Kudos to "Clean Your Plate"!

"*Clean Your Plate* is the self-proclaimed life's work of Author/PhD Amanda Plevell-and it is worth every ounce of effort she put in to it. I read *Clean Your Plate* myself, and the information is amazing. *Clean Your Plate* is an incredibly well-written and knowledgeable book about the connection between the foods we eat and our ability to heal ourselves. However, Amanda herself is the true star of the show. *Clean Your Plate* is truly filled with incredible knowledge. I am a huge fan of this book because it aligns with many of my own holistic health ideas. Honestly, we have a very similar mindset- which I enjoy!"
- Adam Kemp, Professional Basketball Player. Health and Fitness Enthusiast. Holistic Health Advocate, and founder of AdamKempFitness.com

"When I opened the first pages I felt an excitement, a connection with what I believe to be true too. I want to be free from an imprisonment of poor health. I want to have a say in a world where profit often wins. I know the art of eating has become the business of eating. I have been searching for my own health for years! I loved the simple step by step, 1, 2, 3 approach that makes it easy for anyone to begin and to do as much or as little as they are ready for! I loved the community connection and help that each person could tap into in their journey. I was pulled into the book and I kept turning page after page to read how this can help me." - E.N.

"As someone who asks a lot of questions because I like to know the "why/how" behind things, I found this book about food to be very enlightening! The easy to follow along explications of how food is grown, harvested and prepared and how that affects our bodies was so helpful to me!"

"Where it says, "Every time you eat, you are either feeding your body for health or disease" was a powerful reminder!"

"This book encourages you to really pay attention to what you put in your body and observe how it makes you feel/perform."

"What you take in today, determines our body and health tomorrow!'
Thanks for the knowledge and freedom of health provided amongst these pages!!!

"I will be buying copies for all of my loved ones!"   - S.R.

"Very few people view food as fuel for the body, they eat because it tastes good." I feel way better when I stick to clean eating. I've stayed away from boxed food for six months now. It makes a difference!" - B.M.

"Oh my goodness, I love this!" - F.S.

" I love that it tstates '4 steps'...It gives it an un-intimidating feel." - K.H.

"I appreciate that this book is written in layman's terms. This book will be able to help people with breaking the food pyramid fallacy and understanding the food chart and the foods that are essential." - A.S.

"I am able to exercise and make it through a class, my energy is back up, the fogginess and sick feeling is gone! I am sleeping like a rock and not so tired in the morning, I have even been waking before my alarm. And I don't feel as anxious and overwhelmed. I have noticed that the stiffness in my body is gone." - L.N.

"I just wanted to thank you. I was skeptical at first, not so much now. Being able to make a conscious choice and based on that choice being able to recognize the benefits and consequences is very empowering. Your work is amazing and I am thankful that we have crossed paths." - M.M.

"I'm on day 7 of a new understanding of my diet. I want to say a big huge THANK YOU! I am finally starting to feel like myself again, and enjoying life with my family. Yesterday, instead of napping the day away, I had the energy to go out with my husband. I am so grateful for your wisdom and help!"
- A.L.

"I love this! We should fuel our bodies for alertness and success with foods packed with vitamins!" - S.R.R.

"I have never thought about food in the way that I think about it now. I didn't realize what I know now. I always KNEW I wanted to be healthier, I just didn't have the ability to stick to it. This has made all the difference because "Clean Your Plate" has helped me understand that it's not about depravity. The 70/30 image helps me to stay in balance instead of constantly feeling less than and worthless for not being able to stick to a diet. That was only PART of the equation, but changing this image was a big one for me." - E.N.

Clean
Your
Plate

4 Steps to Boldly Empower
Yourself to Create Free Healing
in 5,6,7,8….

Amanda E. Soulvay Plevell, PhD

Published by: Flight Plan Publishing

Clean Your Plate

Amanda E. Soulvay Plevell, PhD

ISBN: 978-1719045742

Published by:
Flight Plan Publishing, MN

Flight Plan Publishing's books and publications are available through most bookstores. For further information, email: info@cleanyourplatebook.com

Clean Your Plate

Amanda E. Soulvay Plevell, PhD

DEDICATION

I dedicate this book to the most important people in my life -
My husband, Jason, and my boys: Evan, Kaden, and Dash,
without whose constant food preferences/particularities, and my desire for
them to eat healthy, this book probably would not have been written.

I also dedicate this book to those who know the struggle of illness and are
returning to a state of the natural to heal. Blessings to you of health and light
on your journey! The body is innately designed to be healthy!

This book is also dedicated to those who dare to be different, who desire to
create something better where it wasn't before, and who dare to defy status
quo in order that truth and integrity prevail. To those bold enough to want to
make a difference not only for themselves, but in order to better the world.

Clean Your Plate

Amanda E. Soulvay Plevell, PhD

CONTENTS

Clean Your Plate

WARNING! THIS BOOK CONTAINS FREE HEALING INSIDE!
READ NO FURTHER IF YOU WANT TO STAY THE SAME!

This is one of the most important books you'll ever read. In a world where it can often seem that much is beyond our control, and many authorities make decisions for us, food and what we put into our bodies is still our choice. Food and our approach to it is HEALING!

No matter where you are in your life right now, we do have one thing in common: we want to be better or you would not have picked up this book. You want to improve your SELF and your expression out into the experience of this world. Whether you are overweight, underweight, struggling with disease, or perfectly healthy, we all eat. We all are bombarded with the same messages and innuendos about what is acceptable , conventional, and "normal", despite the fact that we KNOW the Standard American Diet is severely lacking, and extremely highly disease promoting. We KNOW something must be done, but we are bombarded with corporate funded messages that serve as education, misleading advertising, and the latest and greatest health protocol.

Besides, EVERYONE ELSE eats anything they want, why shouldn't we, right? Wrong. It's not true. Behind every smiling face is a struggle you know nothing about. And it makes no sense to try to figure it out, just to understand EVERY person does struggle you know NOTHING about. Knowing this, how can any one person judge what is right or wrong? We ALL want to be better. Work on YOU. Be a better, stronger, healthier YOU with what makes sense to and for you.

I believe we want to be free from an imprisonment of disease and poor health. I believe we want to have the say over the expression of our bodies, but in a world where profit often wins, we are misinformed and what is NOT WORKING in order to have a healthy body has become what's "normal".

This book is my baby, born of years of professional experience, education and trial and error. It is what I believe to be true over everything I have studied, wrapped up in a way that is user-friendly. It is not the ONLY truth, or the only way to do things, but I've worked hard to extract truth where I've found it in an effort not to propose yet another "diet plan", but real truth about putting you back in the driver's seat of your own health.

To this end, I would like to say that it works for everybody, but you either are ready or you are not. And the fact remains that if you want to continue consuming quarter pounders and downing gallons of soda, I can't morally and responsibly tell you it's going to work for you. To the extent that this information DOES work for everyone is that I believe every person can take even a small part as a step in the right direction. Look to find the place where YOU can start.

I believe we were born with an innate desire to matter, to make a difference, the least of all to ourselves and to our families, and what is surprising to some is that HOW WE EAT makes a difference to our planet and the people on it, from sustainability and health of the planet to the rapid and rising costs of healthcare, insurance, and the impact that has on the taxpayer. We were born with an innate desire to be healthy and happy. Even when others set the stage, we still get to decide in which to take part. It is said whoever controls the food controls the world. I believe this to be true. If you want to take your health and your impact on the planet into your own hands, then it's time to learn about food, unlearn conventionalism, and instead accept what is true, real, and what really works.

As an author, speaker, trainer, and natural health practitioner and coach, my work is focused on helping people take all 8 Dimensions of their life and bring as much fulfillment and happiness as possible. I believe that when we better ourselves, we better our entire world, AND that it is ESSENTIAL that we do this. It is NECESSARY for each of us to discover our Greatness Within and spread it out into the world. I believe you absolutely MUST fuel your body with REAL NOURISHMENT if you want ANY of these dimensions of your life to be successful. You MUST fuel your body with what it was made to function with for EVERY kind of health, including physically, emotionally and mentally. The body needs the right fuel. Just as you wouldn't fuel a diesel engine with 87 Octane, the body has specific fueling needs also. The problem is we all KNOW this, at least intellectually, but DOING it is another thing! Also, we don't have a clear understanding WHY our bodies need certain foods, just that we're told what to eat and what

Amanda E. Soulvay Plevell, PhD

not to eat without a clear understanding of why. I believe that as evolving human beings we don't WANT to be told what to do anymore. We are WELL BEYOND the ineffectual dictatorial and authoritative approaches. We don't just "do as I say" anymore. I believe evolved human beings WANT to know facts and truth so they can make decisions for themselves.

This is not a book on sensationalism. It is meant to give a truthful account of the science behind our food, what functions foods play in our bodies, what makes up a "food", and how to use food effectively so that you can make effective choices about what you want your health outcome to be, rather than to accept current status quo.

I wrote this book as a partner book alongside our new book, "Beyond the Plate" in order to illustrate effectively that the physical understanding of proper nourishment (the how to) is part of the equation. The second part is WHY doing it is so hard and what we can do about it these faulty concepts behind why we eat the way we do. I feel there are two parts to this venture in empowering your free will and choice for health. This book contains the education to physically do that. Its partner book, "Beyond the Plate", discusses the second huge and equally important aspect: your RELATIONSHIP with and concepts about food. You will see some of the same information covered in both books as the basic understanding of food is important to the relevance of the application.

In every food choice we make, we are casting our vote, sending the message to the powers that decide the outcome. Every time we buy that canned, bagged or boxed processed food, we are turning over our authority to the providers of those products, choosing the fate of our health, possibly by accepting the will of false propaganda, and giving away our power to choose.

For those whom are already suffering the effects of disease, food is FREE HEALING! Why wouldn't we employ the nourishing and medicinal benefits of the food properties, ESPECIALLY if we understand which functional foods to eat!? More so than that, food is to be FUEL, the health before healing is needed. If we ate intentionally for our bodies' best benefit, we often times wouldn't need the "healing" that disease necessitates.

I fully believe food is our natural way to an existence void of health complications. I fully believe food is our key to enjoying life and healing many of our chronic complaints including even depression and anxiety, two areas of which are more and more frequently being diagnosed and medicated for.

We have put the power of our lives and our health in the hands of decision makers that have often put the interest of profit and success as their greatest motive though it has and may have ill effect on the interest, health, and safety of the people. No matter what those decisions have been, however, it is still up to US to make the choice. No one can go stomping their muddy boots around in your healthy life unless you let them. It's time to gain control over our most powerful deciding factor: our food.

It is my mission to help people out of personal health imprisonment brought on by confusion and misinformation and into a life of health freedom naturally induced by a lifestyle of good dieting.

Please understand, this book is not written with the focus on any particular disease and is not a substitute for medical advice. This is merely a source of information for you and should be used as a cohesive effort alongside what your particular body needs.

Also, this book is for all styles of eaters. It doesn't "take away" but balances your current efforts so health can be had by all. When you feel like you just don't know where to turn, who to believe, or what to listen to, we return to a state of origination; a basic state of simply understanding the purpose of food, what food is, and how its function in our bodies has the ability to create the health freedom we desire. When we are OUR best, everyone and everything else will benefit, truly changing the whole world, not the least of which, yours.

In Health and Greatest Abundance of Blessings,

Amanda E. Soulvay Plevell, P

"LET FOOD BE THY MEDICINE, AND MEDICINE BE
THY FOOD"
-HIPPOCRATES

****

"TELL ME WHAT YOU EAT, AND I'LL TELL YOU
WHAT YOU ARE"
-ANTHELME BRILLAT-SAVARIN

****

"FOOD IS OUR COMMON GROUND;
A UNIVERSAL EXPERIENCE"
-JAMES BEARD

Clean Your Plate

A Special Invitation

Readers, fans and followers of Clean Your Plate, 7D Nourishment and the Fresh Fridge Formulas make up an amazing camaraderie and council of like minded individuals, all bent on fulfilling the wholism of the self, the least of which through diet.

As the creator and author of "Clean Your Plate", and as a Natural Health Practitioner for the last 12 years, I felt it was an absolute necessity to create a place where readers and followers could connect, support each other, swap recipes and stories about what works for them. I had no idea how explosively supportive it would become. I'm continuously astonished at the amazing help that individuals have been able to provide for each other through this community. They say nothing is new under the sun, that even when it doesn't seem like it, someone, somewhere, has experienced what you're currently going through. All it takes is to ask, reach out, or read what others are facing to learn for yourself.

Simply go to www.facebook.com/cleanyourplate5678 and like our new page. You'll immediately connect to others just like you, working to find a better way to eat and live. You'll find people just beginning and you'll find people that have been following healthy eating for years. Either way, you'll be able to bounce notes and ideas off of each other to accelerate your success.

I also wanted to create a place where the education, self growth and empowerment can continue to grow, so people can take their steps as they are ready. DrFoodie.live is our online toolkit, designed to help individuals find health freedom through food and finding themselves. This site is jam packed full of ideas, articles, lessons, courses, and instructional trainings to ignite your evolution. Please check back often as new material is added daily.

If you'd like to connect with me on social media, visit www.facebook.com/DrFoodielive. Please feel free to send me a direct message or leave a comment.

Clean Your Plate

Introduction

From "Incurable Disease" To Vibrant Health

You'll find that those of us in any sort of wellness profession often do so because of personal health experiences and challenges. We all have incredulous stories of pain and trauma resulting in miraculous stories of healing. My story is no different, and it became the entire reason why I am in the field I love today, doing work I feel is my calling, with a passion for which is desperate in my belief in its necessity for our human lives.

I allowed myself to heal naturally from a place of a very dire state in my health through a discovery of food, stress, balance, some amazing mentors, and resetting my image on life and my limiting belief set, and God.

I am not in the medical field, and serve no place in using this book or any of my work to substitute for professional care and none of this should be construed as medical advice. I do however, want to share truths I have experienced.

My intention is always to increase the good, to bring necessary and useful change, to evolve and grow and to help others to do the same. How people live, our understandings, our thoughts, concepts, and beliefs are hugely interesting to me as I study and research further the field of cellular biology, functioning, quantum energy, and nutritional biochemistry.

Through it all: my education at the natural health colleges I chose, all this research, studying, and my own health experiences have created the way I operate today, both personally and professionally.

Food has become something I inevitably find myself involved in no matter which way I turn. There are extreme disturbances and injustices in my opinion, surrounding the nature, the production, the lies and false propagandas of the food industries and our health practices. Add to that our own demands as humans and we continue a rotting cycle of breeding disease into humanity and the planet we all share. I believe that because it is the center point of so much of our lives, and because of its mass misunderstanding as fuel for our bodies, food is the number one way we can grab hold and empower our own health and lives once again.

I applaud all that pick up this book in an effort to improve life for themselves, because it ultimately affects more than you alone. And to those that are willing to take this information and use it to amass change on the largest platforms available to you, I am supremely thankful.

I encourage you all, individuals, and professionals, to share all the positive changes you experience with everyone you know, and also to us. Feel free to leave me a message anytime at: info@cleanyourplatebook.com.

Amanda E. Soulvay Plevell, PhD

-1 -

THE POWER TO TAKE YOUR HEALTH BACK

I don't think anyone can argue against the fact that what we eat affects our health, either negatively or positively. When over 678,000 each year are related to obesity or nutrition, it seems obvious we need to rethink our conventional diets.

Poor food quality and intake has become an epidemic in our country! Obesity, heart disease, and diet related illnesses are on the rise with no scope of slowing down. Without using our food for healing, but continuing to consume synthetic and man made convenience foods, the problem will simply keep the vicious cycle going.

Continuous new diet fads and trends coming out serve to offer up a platter of conflicting information. We know we are supposed to eat fruits and vegetables, but for convenience sake and availability, the canned, processed choices are little better than the alternative. Worse yet, one can pretty much find studies for both sides saying on either side that these foods can be helpful or harmful to our health. For instance, even the American Heart Association, seen as a trusted resource by many, put out a conflicting article stating how Coconut Oil is "bad" for you![1] No wonder we have gotten off track, when the authorities that we've grown accustomed to listening to send confusing messages as well, and to what (or who's) gain?

We know that the ART of eating has become the BUSINESS of food, and that many stand to profit from our ignorance and

[1] Food Babe. "Is Coconut Oil Healthy? The Controversy Explained." Food Babe, 7 Feb. 2018, foodbabe.com/coconut-oil-healthy-controversy-explained/.

misunderstanding.

Living, also, in a time where the future is uncertain; where access to our nourishing plant medicines, homeopathy, vitamins and supplements can be threatened; where convention dictates where we receive our health care; where more and more processing and alteration is done creating more and more dead foods; and with powers of authority making our healthcare decisions for us...one thing remains. As Hippocrates said, "Let food be thy medicine." As long as we know the functional capacities of food, and make conscious decisions about what we take into our bodies, we have the ability to make the call over the condition of our bodies and its representation of health.

As Hippocrates said, "Let food be thy medicine."
As long as we know the functional capacities of food, and make conscious decisions about what we take into our bodies, we have the ability to make the call over the condition of our bodies and its representation of health.

There are many diets, methods, theories, and misinformation concerning our diets and it can be confusing and overwhelming. When we stop to consider the very simple laws that come into play, hopefully we will have a more clear cut view on how to nourish our bodies healthfully.

My Personal Account

Over the years, I was hit with a plethora of medical complications that have added fuel to my fiery passion for truth and health. These incidences have given me ample opportunity to discover true health and move away from conventional thinking in favor of one that suits the benefit of my body.

My diagnoses included "incurable" disease names, to which I am no longer imprisoned. I do not regret these experiences, because it helped me create an education that is second to none based on having been there. How I work with my clients now comes from true understanding in relationship to their current experience.

I also sustained Steroid Induced Myopathy brought on by commonly prescribed steroidal medication. This put me in a wheelchair, not knowing if would ever walk again, followed by two years of recovery and re-learning how to walk. This is not to spread fear and mistrust of needed and valuable medical systems at the times where they are indeed needed, but to raise awareness that the role food and food medicines play is essential, where I had no knowledge of it before my health disturbances. This is my attempt to share from my experience. Please do make use of every method that is available and makes sense for you at the time it is needed. My intention here is to share what I learned about truth in nourishment and why healthful intake should be a daily habit.

It really is about keeping it simple. Once you understand food and its purposes in the body, it's easier to decide what and when to eat rather than relying on the newest fad diet.

As any good dancer or musician knows, the instructor sets the tempo and preps you for what's coming by shouting out, "and 5,6,7,8!" And off you would go.

In this book we'll go over:

- The FIVE questions to ask yourself before you eat ANYTHING
- The SIX words that make meal planning a snap
- The 7D Nourishment program that pulls it all together for healthy wellbeing
- the 8 Dimensions of Life that you're doing all this for anyway!

Well, here we go, the "and" portion before we count off!

There is More to Food Than Eating

Try as we may, there is an undeniable connection between our food and our health. We can't deny it; it is what makes us up, after all. Trying to have special diets and focus on fad foods of the day serves only to distract us away from the simplicity of the function that food really is: to nourish our bodies with its consumption, and to nourish our soul with the time spent growing, preparing and sharing a meal with the people in our families and communities.

It is equally ignorant to keep moving on in the direction of synthetic pharmaceutical medications as our go-to "healers" when the very reasons for needing those medications haven't been addressed. An objection of those conventionally accepted ideas means we learn to work with intention rather than with an uninformed mentality that simply follows the crowd.

It is important that we are making the vote in favor of our health, our freedom and independence every day, by returning to a state of self-love in order to make good, strong, and healthy decisions over our lives. It is important to use these qualities to say no to the conventionally accepted ideas and beliefs about food that are harmful to us. It is important to use these qualities to say yes to re-learning real food and what it does for our bodies, and how to use it to breed health and clarity of mind. This gives us knowledge and the power over us is back in our hands. This gives us independence from powers of authority that can determine the quality of composition of foods available to us, and the types of medicines we receive. It gives us freedom from negative thought patterns that keep us in a state of not-enough-ness and incompletion, and thus the desire to look outside of ourselves for happiness. It gives us the wisdom to know which foods to eat when, which herbs and plant medicines are here to fortify our bodies, and which to use to support our bodies natural processes.

We need to examine why we've made it so difficult and how to get back to the basics, learning to enjoy the most essential part of our body vehicle's existence.

* To build a relationship to the food we partner with to build our bodies.
*To understand that what we eat today DOES become what we are tomorrow.

*We need to see food as a healer for every part of life.

*That its choice can bring peace and purpose.

*That working with food together and taking time for meals and preparation can bring better relationships with ourselves and with others.

*That it can improve our children, that they will have better health and less medications along with better behaviors.

*That we ourselves will be more stable in our hormones and emotions.

*That we will not only have better health, but a clearer brain, strength and power over our health, and the say in what dictates that outcome.

*That feeling better and more connected in general, will bring us a feeling of being okay.

*That feeling better and less hopeless will bring a sense of unity and the desire to share this with others.

*That respect for what we put into our bodies, the understanding that all people do the very same thing,: eat; and that the earth provides this for us through our efforts brings a continuity and power in the joy of working together.

*A respect and understanding for the cycle of life, which at its very core, starts and ends with providing food for each other.

Food Unites Families, Communities, and Humanity

At the very core, food has always been what brought us together… in times of sorrow, in times or joy and celebration, as well as meals prepared and taken together during the day. If you think about it, the very labor that occupied people's every waking day was in the preparation of food, from farming, plowing, planting, harvesting, storing, canning and preparation, most of the day was spent supporting our nutrition intake.

In every culture, effort has historically been made that groups of people prepare food together. This fast food mentality of ease and convenience is only more and more common since the age of industrialization fifty years ago.

Growing food together, providing for each other's needs, sharing recipes, and gathering to support our neighbor, even as it meant GETTING

TO KNOW THEM, provides for a sense of community and an ethic that it takes a village.

If we want health and humanity, a sense of peace and tolerance over differences, we need again to unite at the very core of what is necessary to our body's' health, and essential to the continuation of Earth itself.. food.

Why Do We Eat, Anyway?

Every living organism requires food for its use. Even the simplest vegetable cell takes in and uses nourishment. Guided by a power we cannot see, the plant takes in, absorbs and uses food that is essential for its growth and development. If given what it needs to survive and thrive, it blooms into a beautiful plant. If, however, it is grown in dry undernourished soil, the plant that will develop will be sickly. We are no different. The nourishment our bodies need in order to survive and thrive is very specific. We need to take an account of the foods available and offered to us currently. Just because it exists does not mean it is beneficial to our Life and/or bodies. Just because fast food exists does not mean it has been passed through and been approved of by a board certification committee that qualifies food establishments for quality nourishment. It exists. It is our power of choice and free will to determine with reason what we will and will not nourish our bodies with. The faulty misconception is that there is a governing organization that looks to the offerings of food available and examines their nutrient content for health. Time and time again food has been discovered to show very negative health consequences, and yet they exist, with the argument that it is our right to choose. In fact, our demand for the freedom of choice can have some very dire consequences when we are also then not taking the time to properly educate ourselves on what is appropriate to eat. It is much easier to be convenient, feed our insatiable need for instant gratification, and stay blind, assuming someone else is watching out for us. It's not true.

It has been said, "He who controls the food controls the world." And that is true. It is one need alongside water, that, if removed, becomes all we would suddenly focus on finding.

Where Have We Gotten Off Track?

We know that from wherever it began, people feel very lost, not sure who or what to trust. Many feel that people are just not taught a foundational education about food any more. Who is doing the teaching? When parents are occupied elsewhere, are worn out, don't bother, don't have time, or don't really even know what the truth is anymore. Parents themselves have to have a good relationship with food in order to pass it down to their kids. Keep in mind, however, that many adults don't have a relationship with food either.

Think, also, on the common responses adults give to WHY they don't teach fundamental healthy food knowledge to their kids. They have chronic fatigue, feel too busy, don't feel well, are stressed, anxious, and/or depressed and convenience is too easy. It is difficult to encourage healthy habits even if you did know them, when you don't feel well. They, too, can want only what makes them instantly and immediately feel good, even if the long term consequences don't manifest health. It is commonly felt there isn't time to worry about those consequences when we barely have time to deal with what's in front of us RIGHT NOW. Thus, we allow children to be like us, because we haven't found our own way out. How can we possibly teach it to them?

We also have allowed the term "food" to encompass foodstuffs and fillers that are in no way nourishing to all use the same title. There is a major difference between a "nourishment" and a "filler", most of which are what our store shelves are supplied with. If you remember, grocery stores never even used to be common place. It should say something about our reliance on them and our lack of obtaining fresh natural foods by the fact that each of us has to "grocery shop".

When it comes to knowing who or what to listen to, do we trust our doctors, organizations, schools ,and our government establishments, or that our parents know what to impart to us? The suggestion could be backed that when it comes to our own health, learning to listen to our own bodies, re-learning the basic function of food and its purpose in our bodies, being mindful of where food comes from, and then being smart and logical as to whether it should be consumed or not, would take us far on our journey away from stress and confusion towards health and peace. It is, after all, only food. The problem, however, is that we are disconnected to our own bodies. There is much to learn about the process of food, and listening to our own body's innate sense of knowledge and guiding force.

Food, real food, grown from the earth and full of nutrients, prepared with natural processes, was originally made for our use, and much to our surprise, still is, without the need of factories and plasticization. Consider it. Your food goes into your body and metabolically breaks down to join your cells. And your cells make you up. Everything you become is what is in the cells to do. And everything that is in the cells to do is made from what you feed them. Every time you eat you are either feeding health or feeding disease.

Every time you eat you are either feeding health or feeding disease.

The purpose of this book is NOT to tell you cannot have certain foods. It is to tell you how you can; when and how to do it appropriately, while still working in favor of the body's health, in a balance that doesn't allow an environment for disease to thrive. It's to teach you HOW to live a "normal" social life, but still vote for your health. Eventually, we hope to re-evaluate the acceptance of "foodstuffs" vs. real food as the "norm". For now, its to demonstrate how food shapes and creates your experience of health or "dis-ease".

If you are already experiencing disease in the body, yes, it will take some time for the blueberries and juiced nutrient supplements to work. For the salads and whole grains to make a difference. Of course, you'll actually start experiencing benefits and symptom relief immediately as your body is able to function better. Over time, as the body's cells rebuild new and healthier uninflamed cells, more and more benefits will be noticed.

Let's begin by taking a look at the basic principles of food, and why on earth we eat in the first place.

Is it Food?

The very nature of food is that nature IS food. There is a drastic variance between what is original food for the nourishment and functioning of the body and what is believed to be food based on what is presented in our stores today. Just because it exists on store shelves and is for sale, and can be ingested by the body does NOT make it food. However, this is the common belief among the population today. Seemingly, we need to go back and have an agreement on the definition of "food".

If it can be ingested, is it food?
If it "tastes good" is it food?
If it fills the belly, but doesn't necessarily nourish the body,
is it food?
If it does not contain a good amount of nutrients in the labeling
is it food?
If it is boxed, canned, processed from its original form, is it food?
If it contains chemical and synthetic ingredients, is it still food?
If it is genetically modified, is it food?

It would do us well to understand the functions that are necessary for the body to perform so that we can understand the PURPOSE of why we eat, before we can then go one to define what is and is not a food.

The Function of Food and The Purpose of Eating

In order to think about the original purpose of food, think first about the body itself. There is a need within the physical body to have energy to serve its other functions. I think we have forgotten that FOOD is what becomes the body. What you eat today determines how strong the muscles will be, how the hair will grow, how the organs will function. In our very inadequate education of food it is not emphasized enough that WHAT WE TAKE IN TODAY DETERMINES OUR BODY AND HEALTH TOMORROW.

Without fuel, the cells don't have energy to convert for the body's use. Without the right kind of fuel, the kind that contains nutrients that turn "energy" into "building blocks", the body doesn't build, grow, transform, or remove its dead cells. Essentially, the process of cellular metabolism (the process of taking in, making use of, and wasting out food substance) doesn't happen. The rest of the body's cells, tissues, and organs would not be fed and would eventually die. Therefore the PURPOSE of eating is to receive fuel and nutrients for the body. Not only do we do this to keep the body alive, but it is important to note that the KINDS of fuel the body is provided with determines the HEALTH of the cells we are nourishing. The FUNCTION of the food, then, is to serve the needs of the body. Which brings us back to discussing the nature of food, allowing us to determine the answer to the question, "WHAT IS A FOOD?"

WHAT WE TAKE IN TODAY DETERMINES
OUR BODY AND HEALTH TOMORROW.

The Very Nature of Food

We say "the nature of food" because WHERE did food originally come from? Back before factories and production lines? Where did the factories get the food to model after, or to create from? You got it: nature. Food was grown in nature, and still is. What is essential, beneficial, and the least toxic to our bodies is the food that is grown naturally and originally intended for the body's use. Where did we ever get the idea that packaged, processed and canned or bagged food was suitable anyway? Or did we just go along with status quo because it was easier in our busy lives?

Let's go back to roots and origination of food. Before it was able to be mass produced and transformed into the colorful packaging it is today, food was in the best packaging it could be...the Earth. It was pluckable straight from the trees, or the ground and consumed immediately. This assured maximum nutrient intake as well as the best chance of receiving the enzymes from that food source. Enzymes not only digest our food, but are the catalysts for every other action in the body. Enzymes in food are naturally formed along with the nutrients within that food. Through some unique innate coding, fresh natural food straight from the source and unprocessed contain not only the nutrients it hosts, but also the wherewithal to break down those nutrients so we can use them. This unchangeable and very important fact of nature has seemingly been forgotten, as evident in our drive towards preserved, processed convenience foods.

This very large bit of unchangeable truth has been pushed to the wayside and at our own detriment. Taking foods from their original source, unaltered, was and is still the best sources of nutrition to match the direct functions of our bodies.

As alternative operations came into play, like fire, for example, it changed what was possible with food, but also changed the properties of food. As technology increased, safer, better, more efficient methods were invented. Soon people understood the time that could be saved, and the food that could be saved by using the new technologies. It was not studied, however, about what these new technologies did to the makeup of the food itself, such was the excitement about the money that could be saved. It was not questioned at the time whether the food remained the same, retained its nutrients and enzymes, or not.

The same is true of refrigeration. The ways of preserving food, the manipulations that could be made to food using heat and cold gave new options, new flavors, and new uses for food. The cycle continues further and further that during the course of trying to find the most time saving, efficient, convenient uses available, less and less of the original food exists. For example, if we want to remove the egg from a recipe so that it can store on shelves, the search is on for a substance that provides the same eggy qualities without the worry of preservation or temperature restrictions for safe keeping. And now we have a synthetic alternative. The same is true in every consideration of preserving food longer, making it more convenient, quicker to prepare, less needy of specific storage. Milk doesn't last long even with refrigeration, and so it is homogenized (spun quickly) to integrate the chemistry of the milk so that it doesn't separate and curdle, and enzymes were removed so that it wouldn't "digest" itself too quickly. There was a reason why the natural separation of milk happened; have we forgotten why? Chemical preservatives are added to extend shelf life. Coloring is added to make it look more appealing. More and more alterations are made for the sake of cost and convenience, and less and less of the original food is retained.

Just ask yourself next time you are in the store: "Would I be able to find this food item naturally? Is THIS how it looks in nature?"

Some argue that these alterations are necessary in order to "feed the planet", when in reality, it only takes us further and further away from our own sustainability. They know that once all food is prepared FOR us, we can't do WITHOUT it. We need to consider at what cost to our bodies, our communities, our health and livelihood, and our planet in general have these efforts to be efficient, cost-savvy, and convenient exploited?

Food, real food, what we will call "fresh" food, is natural, and found in NATURE, not because the label says "natural", especially because that very word means different things to different people. What "natural" truly means is that if it is found in nature, able to be picked and eaten with minimal preparation, then it is a real food. The fact that it has a label should be the first flag.

Our vegetation provides our carbs, and our herbs are our medicines. Beans, nuts and seeds are our proteins, as well as any animal products you believe in consuming. The fact of the matter is, what the body needs was and is capable of being naturally created on the earth. It is possible that the more and more our needs are met OUTSIDE of us, the more reliable we are on whatever is produced and unnatural.

So the definition of food for the purposes of this book is " a naturally grown substance taken into the body, that functions to nourish the individual's specific functions, and does not impede or injure these functions."

"Natural" terminology in labeling does not necessarily mean that it is a pure food or product. It could mean that it was made with a portion of products that are know not be grown by nature, but it does not necessarily mean pure, or that it is WHOLLY grown in nature. For example, "natural flavors" means they are FLAVORINGS mimicking natural sources, but not necessarily the source itself.

It can be hard to learn what is real and true in health and wellness since it is such big money, and that is why it is important to listen to your body and keep educating yourself. It is also important to not take things as truth before you've checked into them. Remember that food manufacturers have their own agendas: profits and board satisfaction, to name a couple. Many things are accepted without us looking into them and this is unwise on our parts. Keep in mind just because it exists on a shelf does not mean it is healthy for us. Many foods that are very dangerous for our health are posted right on the product, but few people pay attention to the labeling, or know what it means even if it did. Besides that, "everyone else is buying it" and herd mentality wins again, without even KNOWING what you're eating or where it comes from.

For example: Aspartame is one of those substances that are grossly unhealthy and damaging to our bodies, and is in many many products, and is commonly used and accepted despite the serious and deadly effects. Look at some of its known side effects: cancer, headaches, dizziness, seizures, skin rash, ADHD, learning disorders, weight gain, Alzheimer's, and more. The editorial team at Healthline states, "While aspartame is indeed approved by the FDA, the consumer advocate organization Center for Science in the Public Interest has cited numerous studies that suggest problems with the sweetener, including a study by the Harvard School of Public Health." The fact that any substance is being questioned warrants further study, in my opinion. It's not even hidden from us on the packaging, but the public purchases products containing it anyway. What goes into your body needs to be checked into. No one can be blamed if one has not made knowledge and conscious living a priority.

When it comes to wellness, I believe it is best not to be bogged down by philosophy or creed, but instead to see the results for yourself. Keep things simple and understand there are basic functions playing out in the body and the goal that is well within your hands is to live in such a way that these functions are not impeded, certainly not by the food you fuel them with.

Clean Your Plate

-2-

Zones: The Functions of the Body

Over my time, education, and experience, I have come to develop a love for the study of Biomechanics and Quantum Biomechanics: the function and purpose of life/ the function and purpose of all things and consider it to be a cornerstone of my belief set and teaching style.

I like to follow the approach of zone healing doctors around the nation who were trained in Dr. Thurman Fleet's structuring of the systems of the body. These zones include:

Perfect Digestive Health
Perfect Muscular Health
Perfect Circulatory Health
Perfect Nerve Health
Perfect Eliminative Health
Perfect Glandular Health

Using this "Zone Healing" model, I find it easy for client and practitioner to keep a simple focus on the suggestion of perfect health, and the idea of "functional wellness".

Functional Wellness is the unique term for the natural health practice of identifying the body as a functioning unit containing systems of function comprised of cellular structures serving a function. In layman's terms, everything has a job and a purpose and a reason to be inside of this amazing capsule of the human body. Functional Wellness is not about defining the ailment, illness, or disease by term or diagnosis. It is about taking the body from where it IS to an image of where we want it to BE. Through the process of identifying functions that are imbalanced and thus not allowed to "do their job", supporting the functions of the body cells, systems, and unit as a whole, and imaging wellness the body is returned to a normal state of function.

It is the belief that a person can heal in the microcosm of the body, just as the world can heal in the macrocosm if each individual unit is allowed to perform its purpose and function. That is why I am so intent on helping each person to find out their personal function and purpose, in order to serve the macrocosm and create change for all. Understanding the functions of the physical is just a means to the end...growth, transformation and evolution for all.

I believe in function and purpose in everything. Like a well oiled machine, if we perform our function from the tiniest microcosm of the cell to the individual's service to the purposes of situations, thoughts, and events we see the connectedness that has the potential to ever increase the wellness of our world and everyone in it.

-3-

FOOD AND ILLNESS

What never ceases to intrigue me is both:

1. The healing nature of food, and
2. The complete misunderstanding of it, despite the fact that we know healthy eating reduces risks of illness.

While a large majority of people seem to follow a conventionally accepted commercial and processed diet out of misunderstanding, avoidance, emotion, conventional beliefs, misguided direction, or any other reason, it still amazes me that while food is known to be healing, the amazing risks, schemes, and finances we are willing to expend in order to demand health post poor food decision making is frightening!

More and more people each year are diagnosed with nutritionally related illnesses, or those that could be altered, moderated, or prevented altogether with proper nourishment. Besides that insidious problem, obesity is rising at an alarming rate, particularly among the youngest population. I must say at this point, I do not believe nor engage in a judgemental philosophy, I do not judge people who struggle. We all have stories, reasons, and concepts and about this I believe three things. One, when a flower wilts, you don't blame the flower, you fix the environment in which it is grown. What do we expect with misguided and inadequate education that often does not work towards the good of the people? And if "obesity is a problem, this is the portion of the "problem" I have an issue with. Two, while the PERSON, themselves are not the "problem". The fact that we live in a world that accepts skewed ethics for the sake of profits is. The person is lovable and worthy. Their choices have reasons behind them. However, EVEN THOUGH the above exists, if the person desires improvement, it IS up to them; blaming the system won't help one single person to take charge of their own health; ignorance is not an excuse. ANYONE who wants a healthier life cannot afford to fall back on reasons or excuses if they truly want to improve and this goes beyond obesity to all life in general. What needs to happen is we need to stop writing off people as "obese" and see them instead as people with a history and an explanation. What is a sad fact is that quite commonly, someone with an illness gains sympathy and understanding where someone with obesity is looked at with blame and judgement. If a person is asking for help their history including explanations and concepts need to be examined in order to be effective. The condition should not devalue the person as a whole. I believe all people should have a chance to be able to make true and accurate choices about their health and faulty authoritarian advertisement should not supercede this end goal.

"Obesity rates have climbed to 40 percent and related medical costs are exceeding $147 billion yearly," said Barbara Ainsworth, Ph.D., chair of the American Fitness Index Board and a Regents' professor in the Exercise Science and Health Promotion Program in the School of Nutrition and Health Promotion at Arizona State University."

I find passion in sharing personal experiences for the good of the whole, and when a person IS ready, despite the obstacles, I love watching their faces and their own excitement evolve when they remove hopeless victimization and understand the scope of their own power.

Having said all that, it is pointless, in my opinion, to invest hours on determining "right" vs. "wrong", rather what works and what doesn't work. It is clear that conventional food and dietary practices are not working. This book is an attempt at instituting an easy solution of what DOES work...simple principles that are easy to employ and certainly aren't sugar-coated (pun intended).

Amanda E. Soulvay Plevell, PhD

Why Eating the Blueberry Won't Cure You

With more and more confusion being thrown our way through fad diets, "expert" philosophy and the latest and greatest medical breakthroughs, it's easy to get a skewed conceptual construct when it comes to the ease with which our diet should be. Add to that the fact that there is more mistrust with conventional practices and alternative practices alike, more bias, and less trust with our lawmakers, our manufacturers, our governing agencies, and with who and what we should believe than ever before.

All of these factors have caused us to develop an even weaker understanding of the healing power of food itself. Healing with food is FREE! What we put into our bodies INEVITABLY has to make a difference to our health or the lack thereof. Consuming appropriate, nutrient rich foods and eating them well HAS to, therefore, make positive change one way or another. We search the internet for the magical foods that reduce blood pressure, make us skinny, cure diabetes. Infographics proclaim the benefits of eating blueberries and acai. For a time, we gobble them up and when they don't produce instant benefits, we give up and go back to the Cheetos.

Here is the thing: there are hundreds of foods that will assist the body's healing, that will reduce the symptoms of depression, or of chronic heart disease, or of skin conditions. HOWEVER, the FOOD is not a magic bullet. A FOOD is the necessary FUEL for the body to do what it already knows to do. It's already innately PROGRAMMED to do it. A diesel engine already KNOWS how to run and what to do, now all it needs is DIESEL FUEL. The "blueberry", "acai juice", or "magic secret food discovered in the heart of Africa" is simply the FUEL to allow the programming to happen. The problem is that we have the concept and belief that something on the OUTSIDE needs to come in and TAKE OVER to MAKE the body healthy. We JUST NEED TO GIVE IT THE FUEL IT NEEDS, and that includes eating the healthy variety of fresh foods, unadulterated, unprocessed or minimally processed, CONSISTENTLY EVERY DAY.

Healing INEVITABLY has to happen when the body is allowed to do what it knows to do. This is why "eating blueberries to heal cancer" will never work, because you haven't fully embraced or understand the idea of fueling a functioning system as a PRACTICE, a LIFESTYLE, not as an addition to an already poor diet and a poor relationship to the food that makes up that diet, which is what really needs to change. If you keep the idea that the blueberries are the "healer", while you continue to eat your burger and fries with large soda, you've really only stayed consistent with the mentality that the "pill" will heal your problem, rather than a complete understanding that it takes ALWAYS fueling the diesel engine with diesel fuel EVERY TIME you fill up the tank, not just adding a cleaning substance every once in a while.

Get Out Of The Way

Food is healing, not just in consumption but during the whole process, much of which we no longer take any part of. The body prepares and is just as much a part of the process as eating and digesting the food is. It is not a singular action. Digestion starts LONG before it even passes your lips. The body prepares for intake of nourishment all the time. When it's selecting or choosing its food it is already sending messages to the brain: of what it wants to eat, of what it's going to do with the food once it's in the kitchen, how it will be prepared. The body is already acting on its nutritional needs all the time. Even when you aren't in this moment eating calcium foods, but the body needs it, it is already finding it somewhere in your body and moving it to where it needs it. Or it's planning a craving so that you choose something with calcium, or it's preparing hormones that will respond negatively when it doesn't have what it needs. When you are preparing food, smelling the smells, hearing the sounds, your body is already producing enzymes in preparation for digesting it. Your stomach is already answering the cues to achieve appropriate acidity levels for optimal use of the food.

Your body is already preparing for what it needs to do with the food before it even goes in. Obviously what we put in is going to make a difference to health, as we previously discussed. Not only is healthy food part of the healing process by feeding and nourishing our bodies, giving building nutrients, but it also supports our health by using particular nutrients to heal, rebuild, and carry out toxins and wastes.

Just as there are many processes that are carried out that we give little thought to, there are many properties of our food that are given very little thought as well. Sure, we can classify and organize them into like characteristics as the food pyramid allows us to do, however there is little talk to what function a food plays inside the body. There are many properties of foods that are not commonly thought of by conventional nutrition methods. We know we should eat vegetables, but do we really understand why? Has anyone explained the importance to us? And did you notice that processed foods also fit into the categorizing system of the food pyramid as "real" food? For example: my kids came home from school with WRAPPERS in their pockets from their breakfast. What REAL food naturally comes in wrappers? Sure, the cinnamon sticks qualified as two servings of the "grain group", but their nourishment wasn't figured in at all.

Clean Your Plate

-4-

PRINCIPLES IN NOURISHMENT

Of course what goes on the plate is important, but of even more importance, in my opinion, is what the body DOES with it once it's inside. I use the term "nutrition" to mean the breakdown of the makeup of the intended meal, and "nourishment" to mean the bioavailability, metabolism, and use inside the body. With this understanding anything that does not "nourish" the body has no place IN the body. It does not constitute a real food.

So what is "real" food?

We hear this question repeatedly, so it would be good to know what that means, exactly. Real food constitutes a food that has as minimal processing as possible. It is a natural food grown as clean as possible, without additives and processing, taken from natural environment to plate. It is the foods that were meant to function the body, like fruits, vegetables, grains, seeds, beans, rice, lentils, etc. Some people include "real" food to mean meats and some do not. For our purposes, we are going to use the term "fresh", because we are trying to encompass healthy capacity for all eating styles. For meat eaters, this would mean adding fresh caught fish and clean butchered meats without additives and preservatives to the list of real foods above.

Put simply, boxes, cans and bags of processed, colored, seasoned and flavored foods are not "real". They are not clean, pure and fresh and they include the problematic ingredients that bring inflammation and illness to the body.

We use the term fresh to mean the freshest, closest to nature as possible foods with as little processing as possible, the cleanest and purest forms.

We use the term fresh to mean the freshest, closest to nature as possible foods with as little processing as possible, the cleanest and purest forms.

Fresh foods contain the highest nutrient and enzyme content, all of which are necessary for the body's healthy functioning. Fresh foods are the foods that are the first deleted due to "convenience" and time, when in reality, fresh foods are the easiest to eat fresh from the earth, without much preparation but a quick wash. For example, what's faster than grabbing an apple off the tree and wiping it off?

This is one of the many misunderstandings we have adopted over time that have put us on a path of confusion when it comes to our food.

Food Should Not Have to Be Complicated

Food should not have to be complicated. None of the information in this book is meant to make food hard, just to re-educate based on how the processes work for the body. Pretty simply, healthy eating can be summed up as "eat real foods and mostly plants". Anyone can add more vegetation to their diet.

Recipes are not necessary to create fantastic tasting and healthy meals, in fact, the more involved a recipe is, the more personal processing you are doing to the food. Having said that, it is well noted that food prepared at home is far better than food prepared commercially, even with the amount of personal processing is done, it can never rival what is done in factories.

Food is finest and purest in its most raw form with the least amount done to it to make it safe and available in our bodies. With that in mind, meal planning and preparation becomes easy because it's easy and natural foods.

Keep in mind, however that a transformation or change of lifestyle eating is a baby stepping process. It's a transition period and we need to be forgiving with ourselves. Learning as we go is the best way to do it because it will be applicable to us. Most people in a reset period are coming from a conventional, processed and prepared diet. If we've been eating processed flavor additive foods, it can be hard to switch right to fresh and have it taste good where one is going to stick with it. Plus, many people don't know how to begin making "meals" with healthy recipes that taste good, or at least similar to the foods they've been used to. So taking time to allow your body, your habits, and your taste receptors to improve works to achieve more effective results and you'll see more longer lasting permanent change taking place. Take one meal a day and work to improve it and gradually build on from there, for example. Or, determine to add one green juice every day, even if you change nothing else. Or, make the effort to include two vegetables servings with each protein or grain carb. The Fresh Fridge Formulas in step 6 and the 7D Nourishment plan in step 7 are the best I have come up with, but all steps towards improvement is better than no steps and continuing to blindly accept status quo.

The Law of Nourishment

Every day more and more people search for truth, for a real understanding of life, and for a natural way to improve their health and their own lives.

Understanding this, and also understanding that there could be no healing without teaching, and believing in the natural laws that exist for everyone, a man named Dr. Thurman Fleet set out to educate anyone who was willing to listen about these laws and how to use them to better themselves.

The portion of his work that interests us in the purposes of this book are principles he defined and delineated as the "Law of Nourishment". It is a practical application written in an effort to teach people how to overcome the biases of fads and popularity and instead use principles that don't waver.

I endeavor to continue on with the principles discovered and defined by Dr. Fleet, that all might return to a remembrance of function and purpose in our nourishment and the reasons we eat. Truth never changes and it is with that in mind that we educate on the idea of functional wellness.

The Law of Nourishment identifies functions of food that work to correlate with the very purposes of the body's systems. It is the idea that nourishing the body with functional nutrition in which to support the body systems, is the most logical method of nourishment. Not so much WHAT goes on the plate, but what the BODY does with it once it is consumed.

The Law identifies that every food can fall into at least one category of function: Builder, Congestor, Eliminator, Lubricator. These do not change over time. A protein is a builder is a builder is a builder. It always has and always will build the body. With the understanding that this itself is TRUTH, not because a researcher said so or a study documented it, we can move on to learning how to properly use these functioning foods for the functions of our body. For example, an Eliminator food will help the body to eliminate, so we eat them particularly to help the body's eliminative processes. For example, if one is constipated, they probably need more Eliminator foods in their diet. Congestor foods keep the body properly congested so our blood and other fluids are the right consistency, but when overdone cause too much congestion, for example: sinus congestion, clogged arteries, or constipation. When eaten in balance with each other, the functions balance each other out, providing the body with everything it needs. More information can be learned about the Law of Nourishment by researching the topic itself, Dr. Fleet, or by obtaining the author's previously published book, "Doable: How to follow the Law of Nourishment".

We, however, will move on to study in depth the functions foods present. Not only does each food perform a function, but the order and balance with which these foods are eaten is important as well.

There's an order to everything in the universe, including what you eat, how, when, and what comes first. Have you ever watched movies, or read books where the characters ate their meals in courses? Courses were basically steps to their meal. They ate one thing in the first course, then a second course came with a different food, and so on and so forth. They probably knew something about healthy eating that we don't. They did this because they KNEW salad greens needed to come first, and served a purpose in the boy by doing so.

Following the understanding of functions of food, it would make sense why we would consume certain foods first. For example, if one eats raw eliminators first, one prepares the body and its digestive juices and digestive process to accept the more difficult to digest foods that are coming to follow. These eliminator foods are typically raw fresh greens, rich with enzymes for breaking down the entire meal. Protein foods can be eaten next as the body is prepared to handle, by being enzyme rich, these harder to digest foods. If we study the function of the body, eating becomes about how to serve the function of the body, creating functional and systemic wellness.

Before we can get into steps 5,6,7,8 to boldly empower your health freedom through food, it would behoove us to take a quick step back to understand the 4 Basic Food Functions.

Clean Your Plate

-5-

Food Fx: The Four Food Functions

We're used to categorizing our food according to the food pyramid method. But it would make much more sense for us to categorize our food according to what they do in the body. There is nothing new about these foods, it will just help us to understand their use for our bodies if we group them according to their function in the body. Much of the information in this Food Function section is a sharing of what Dr. Thurman Fleet discovered and recorded, along with my further development of the exploration of these functions. I will forever be grateful for the introduction to a friend and mentor, Dr. Jason Lupkes, D.C., who shared the messages Dr. Fleet delivered that changed my life at a time when I was first facing these "incurable" diagnoses, and beyond.

Dr.Fleet was the first I know of to categorize foods into function. He categorized foods into four basic functions as far as their service to the body:

Builders, Eliminators, Congestors, and Lubricators.

In my opinion, keeping it simple can go far to serve your needs within the body. For example, if you break a bone, you will want to be eating Builders. If you are constipated, you are probably eating too many Congestors. If you have diarrhea, you could add Congestors.

One can also see, when looking at the chart on the next few pages, that within each category there are better options than others. For example, a person who is on a grain free diet, can still eat Congestors that are not grain related and receive that function. Eating molasses is better than cake, for example, and its important to notice which options you are continuously choosing over others.

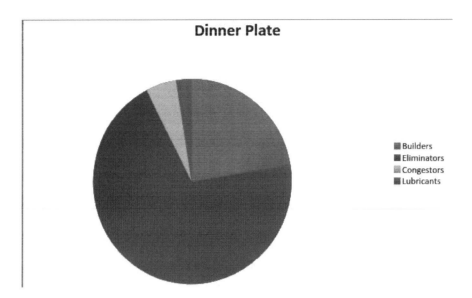

This pie chart illustrates by showing how much of our plate should be made up of each group.

The Builder Food Function: Choose 1 at every meal

These foods build the body. We should not each too much of these foods, as they are acid forming in the body and we want the ph of our bodies overall to be slightly alkaline. Notice the portion of the plate that is reserved for Builders.

We need builders to build all the parts of the body from the cell to the tissues to the muscles, ligaments, bones and skin.

To Be Or Not To Be: Vegan or Vegetarian?

There is much discussion about whether proteins need to come from meat or not. Morality aside, this is a discussion as far as the physical needs of the body. At this time, it is not the intention of being able to label oneself as "vegan" or "vegetarian, but that the protein needs of the body are met to complete the "Builder" function. The discussion then becomes about achieving consumption of all of the amino acids found within protein.

All proteins contain amino acids, of which there are twenty, nine of them being "essential", meaning they must be obtained from the diet, as the body will not produce them. Meat proteins contain all 20, as do plant proteins though in lesser quantities of essential aminos. "In the past, it was believed that people who do not consume animal proteins must combine plant proteins to make up for the missing essential amino acids. For example, since rice is low in the amino acid lysine, but beans are a rich source of lysine yet low in methionine, then a person should eat these foods together to get access to all 20 amino acids. This idea was very popular in the 1970's but questions remain about the importance of protein combining or 'complementary proteins'.. Research now tells us that the body is capable of obtaining the amino acids it needs for health as long as a variety of foods that contain all amino acids are consumed in the diet. A varied diet creates a pool of amino acids the body can use. There is no need to consume all 20 amino acids at each meal, and this idea is now considered irrelevant if you follow a healthful diet."[2]

According to this research and that of many others, it is entirely possible for all protein needs, and "builder" function of the body to be obtained through plants, nuts, and seeds.

Typically, consumers eat far more than necessary from the Builder function, anyway, particularly of meat containing Builders. Dr. Fleet determined that eating one serving of Builders at each meal was and is sufficient.

It is another error on our plates to accept the belief that protein must come from meat sources. Again, if you are vegan or vegetarian, you already know the realm of plant based proteins to choose from, not to mention the protein that comes from vegetables.

---

[2] "Building Complete Proteins from Nuts, Grains and Legumes / Nutrition / Proteins." / Nutrition, www.fitday.com/fitness-articles/nutrition/proteins/building-complete-proteins-from-nuts-grains-and-legumes.html.

Original list of Builder Foods:

Nuts	Avocado	Milk	Eggs
Dried beans	Mushrooms	Lentils	Cheese
butter	Fish	Chicken	Turkey
Beef	Wild Game	All Flesh Foods	

Examples of Plant Based Builder foods:

	per 100g (3.5oz) of weight[3]
Quinoa	4.4
Kidney Beans	4.83
Pinto Beans	4.86
Green Peas	5.36
Macadamia Nuts	7.79
Lima Beans	7.80
Garbanzo Beans	8.90
Lentils	9.02
Pecans	9.50
Soybeans	13.10
Walnuts	15.03
Hazelnuts	15.03
Cashew	15.31
Chia Seeds	15.60
Tofu	17.19
Flaxseed	19.50
Pistachio Nuts	21.35
Almonds	22.09
Hemp Seed	23.00
Peanut Butter	25.09
Pumpkin Seeds	32.97

---

[3] "Vegan Protein." Vinchay Fit Carts, www.pinterest.com

Do you see the error in thinking we need large quantities of meat in order to obtain it? According to the Medline Plus Medical Encyclopedia, the average woman needs 46 grams of protein per day; the average man needs 56 grams per day.[4]

Also, note: This list does not include the protein rich sources in the Eliminator Group. As Eliminator function many protein rich vegetables are included in the Eliminator Group. Win, win!

The Congestor Food Function: Eat sparingly

These foods are the grains, sugars, sweets and starches. They help oxygen to combine with minerals, giving you energy, power, and stamina. Do not eat a large amount of these foods because they cause congestion. Congestion means "stagnant" or "still". Congestion keeps the body from moving bodily fluids and wastes out of the body appropriately. Congestion can cause constipation, belly pains, gas, bloating, nausea, headaches, runny nose, stuffy sinuses, and a heavy chest.

Most people eat too much starch. Think of the things you eat for snack. Are they breads? Crackers? Sugary foods? These are all in the Congestor category and they are typically the foods we reach for because they are convenient, quick to grab and easy to munch on. However, too much starch sets the stage for sinus trouble, constipation, colds, asthma, chest congestion, whooping cough, colitis and other diseases of inflammation and congestion.

Original Congestor Foods List:

Starches: Potatoes, sweet potatoes, all breads, all cakes, macaroni, noodles, spaghetti, flour, gravies, all things made from flour, baked goods, cereals, corn

Sweets: All sugars and sugar substitutes, bananas, pumpkin, squash, honey, molasses, all dried fruits, all candy, all gum, all soft drinks, all canned fruits containing sugar or syrup, jams, jellies, any foods containing sugar or

---

[4] Zieve, D (2009, May 2). In Protein in Diet: MedlinePlus Medical Encyclopedia. http://www.nlm.nih.gov/medlineplus/ency/article/002467.htm

sweeteners including honey, agave, brown rice syrup, molasses, maple syrup, etc.

The Lubricator Food Function: Eat sparingly

This is the group that not only helps to build tissues along with the builders, but it also supports nerve function, brain development and acts as a lubricant inside the body, easing joint movement, and helping the body eliminate wastes.

These are highly fattening foods and can also clog parts of the body if eaten in too great a quantity, so it is best to eat these necessary foods sparingly.

Original Lubricator List:

Butter
Vegetable Oil
Olive Oil
All oils

The Eliminator Function: Choose at least 2 at every meal

This functions contains fruits, vegetables, green leafy and herbs. These foods tear down and remove wastes from the body. They repair tissues and tear down the parts of the body that need to be torn down. These are the "housekeepers" and "trash collectors" of the body and the role they play is very important. It is essential to the health of the body that waste products do not stay inside the body too long. What would happen if there was no one in your home to take out the garbage? What would happen to that garbage? Would you like living there for long?

Most people do not eat enough from the Eliminator category. We need to strive to try new foods, and teach ourselves to like foods from this category. We especially need to eat Eliminators that are green and leafy. Always eat 3 times as much of these foods as the Builders.

Original Eliminator List:

Fruits including: lemons, limes, grapefruits, oranges, pineapples, peaches, cherries, apricots, plums, apples, pears, blackberries, raspberries, strawberries, cranberries, currants, gooseberries, cantaloupe, muskmelon, honeydew, watermelon, tomatoes, and all fruits except bananas

Vegetables including: celery, spinach, endive, lettuce, carrots, asparagus, dandelion, parsley, swiss chard, onions, beets, green peppers, peas, cucumbers, raw cabbage, cauliflower, string beans, artichokes, summer squash, and all other vegetables

I have since added further explanation of the particular functions of fruits, vegetables, and herbs. Within the Eliminator category, there are multiple functions served. Fruits are fast eliminators and are nature's way of protecting the body from potential hazardous pathogens that may have entered the body into the stomach. Fruits help to purge these, being fast eliminators.

Vegetables contain the true carbs to take in for the body. So while vegetables are eliminators, the vegetables also have the carbohydrate energy potential we believe only comes from grain sources.

Green leafy's contain all Eliminator functions.

Herbs are the plant medicines provided for us in nature and are eliminative specifically with medicinal properties of nourishing, cleansing, and removal.

The Eliminators are generally the only Ph alkaline foods among the food function categories. In order to balance and stabilize the acidity from the Builders, Congestors, and Lubricators, double the amount of Eliminators are needed. This illustrates that vegetation should make up the greatest portion of our diet, according to functional wellness.

In order to have proper functioning of all systems, vegetation should make up the greatest portion of our total dietary intake. The macronutrients:

proteins, fats, and carbs are discussed almost incessantly in the nutrition and fitness realms, however, receiving these macronutrients from vegetation, or plant based food sources is much less discussed, as is their animal and grain sourced counterparts. Macronutrients can also be entirely received through plant sources.

According to the 2018 Fitness Index, only "30% of adults reported eating at least two servings of fruit per day, while only 18% indicated eating three or more servings of vegetables per day"

Vegetation has taken everything into consideration when it comes to providing for every system in our body, including the waste removal system, with a plan for clearing toxins out of the cells and then out of the body. Every need for the nervous system to get messages to the brain has been thought of with vegetation, and every need for problem substances in the body to be cleared has been thought of with vegetation. Every energy need has been thought of through vegetation, and every "medicine" need any time the body needs to ramp up its efforts and get assistance from food to clear harmful pathogens, bacterias, fungus, and parasites has been thought of through vegetation.

All vegetation acts as eliminative as its top function, with additional functions depending on the type of vegetation. For instance, green leafy vegetation act as Eliminators, tone the nervous system, remove toxins and benefit hormones and the entire endocrine system. Fruits are fast eliminators and serve a great purpose in quickly eliminating negative products from the body, and feeding the body's quick sugar needs. There is a whole other category within the vegetative world that gets little attention other than for culinary uses: herbs and other plant greens. These are the natural "medicines" to be consumed daily. I hesitate to call them "medicines" because definitely they are known to have medicinal properties, but concepts around the term of "medicine" suggests that a disease, illness, or symptom is present FIRST and then a "medicine" is taken to remove it. In the true understanding of healing food and vegetation, we need to understand that these foods of course are used as such in the form of "herbal medicines" but more importantly, these foods should be consumed daily not as a "preventative" but as the necessary actions to setting the stage for "health".

It is important to instill a concept of understanding the function and purpose of this category of healing foods. The function is NOT as a preventative, though that it does, we don't eat them in order to "prevent" anything. If that is the concept that is being constructed, then the negative concept (that we need to prevent disease) is still present. The concept is still present in the construct of the cells and builds with the idea that we are victims over disease. When, instead, you eat, with a picture of pure perfect health for the sake of it, the cellular constructive blueprint changes. You aren't "fighting" anything, at the whim of anything as a victim, but as a knowledgeable chooser in setting up the environment for the body to build itself, heal itself, and take care of itself using the functional foods that were exactly designated to do so.

When you don't use food as food is meant to be, as fuel for the cells to become the parts of the body, there is no need for the digestive processors, enzymes and chemicals that give the food taste and function to be productive any longer. There is no need for the stimulus of the nervous system to activate these. Without the foods to extract our nourishment from and continue to build a body that carries on, and without that necessary stimulus of the nervous system, much of the natural "body electric" is diminished. You may have heard this to be called CHI. And while there are many ways for the body electric to weaken, it is crucial to note that this weakens both the ENERGY of the body field AND the PHYSICAL form of the body.

To get back into a state of health, functional wellness must be observed, which involves a return to a state of wellbeing. A WELL being naturally has a higher energetic vibration than that of a SICK one.

Dr. Fleet made a chart to represent these four basic food functions. Over the years, I have added to it to include further explanation. I keep a full chart on my fridge and in my office, as well as a blank chart with which to chart our daily meals to teach balance to my kids and clients, as well as to do mini check ups on our dietary balance. If we strictly follow the Fresh Fridge Formula you will learn in the next chapter, we don't need to chart as food functional balance is already accounted for within the formulas.

Food Functions

BUILDERS	ELIMINATORS ☆	CONGESTORS	LUBRICATORS
• Eat after eating raw elimination • Step 2	• Eat raw before anything • Eat also with meal • Steps 1 and 2	• Eat at end, only if still hungry • Step 4	• Eat along with meal • Step 1
• BUILD BODY	• TEAR DOWN • REPAIR • ELIMINATE WASTE • 3 KINDS • ENZYME RICH	• ALLOWS OXYGEN TO BE USED DURING ENERGY RELEASE	*LUBRICATE JOINTS * JOB'S * BRAIN AND TISSUES *CELLULAR SHIELD *NERVE SHIELD-MYELIN SHEATH
1 FOR EACH MEAL	2 FOR EACH MEAL NO MORE THAN 3 FRUIT SERVINGS/DAY	SPARINGLY AT EACH MEAL	USE AS NEEDED
Avocados Beans Beef Butter (also lubricator) Cheese Eggs Fish Fowl Lamb Lentils Milk Mushrooms Nuts Pork	Fruits All fresh fruits except for bananas No more than 3 servings per day *NO CANS! Vegetables: All fresh vegetables Garden canned vegetables Frozen Vegetables Cruciferous *NO CANS! Greens and herbs: All fresh greens(ex.) Beet tops Dandelion Greens Parsley Cilantro Kale Spinach Mustard Greens Collard Greens Turnip Greens Celery Greens	All candy All cereals All gum All soft drinks Anything made from flour All breads Anything made from grains Bananas Honey Corn Dried Fruit Potatoes Bread Cake Flour Gravy Jams Jellies Macaroni Molasses Noodles Noodles Rice Crackers Cookies	Butter All oils All fats Use: Sunflower oil Walnut oil EV olive oil Coconut oil (endures heat)
ph +	ph -	ph +	

How to Chart Your Meals With Food Functions

One method I use repeatedly with clients is to chart what they're eating, right on the food function chart. By adding a tally for each food eaten in it' appropriate column, two purposes are accomplished:
1. It allows a person to instantly notice imbalances among the functions
2. Correcting those imbalances is made simple, by showing how you can eat what you choose, but what you need to add to create balance.

Meal Charting Example:

If the meals of the day are:
Breakfast: 2 cups of cereal with milk and a banana(shown on the first line)
Lunch: 2 slices of bread with turkey sandwich(shown on the second line)
Supper: roast beef with potatoes and corn(shown on the third line)

The chart would look like this:

Builders	Eliminators	Congestors	Lubricators
		lll	
l		ll	
l		ll	

Line one represents breakfast. One tally for each cup of cereal, one for banana(though a fruit, it is not eliminator function. With 6 tbsp of sugar in each one, it qualifies as a congestor)
Line two represents lunch.
Line three represents supper.

Do you see how this particular person did not eat anything "bad" per se, But when looked at according to function, it is heavily imbalanced, using only ph acidic functions.

Correcting the Imbalance

To correct the imbalance, this individual could balance breakfast by reducing cereal to one cup, adding 1 cup of sliced berries, and a handful of nuts on top, and one glass of juice.

Or, reduce cereal to one cup, add a slice of toast, with 2 tbsp of peanut butter, a cup of berries, and a glass of juice.

For lunch she could add lettuce and tomato to her sandwich, and a side salad.

For supper, even though she was eating vegetables, she did not know they served a Congestor function, reducing the meat and Congestor serving and replacing with 2 servings of vegetables would serve to balance this meal.

You can watch meal charting videos on our youtube channel: DrFoodie Amanda Plevell - YouTube.

-6-

The Science of Food

Food, Chemistry, and Energy

We've discussed what makes up a "food", the functional categories they fall into and the functioning systems of the body. Now let's talk about how it all works together.

What we put into our bodies is important. If you are in science class, and you are doing some chemistry experiments, you will mix different components together and see a variety of different reactions. Some can even explode when mixed together. Our bodies are like that chemistry beaker: we should not expect that we can put any substances that we want in there, especially those void of the intended makeup of components that were meant to work together, and not expect some explosive reactions to happen. When we do that, we notice symptoms like gas, bloating, and heartburn because they are immediate. What we may not link together are other symptoms, because they may often be delayed, much longer after the ingestion of food and we may miss the correlation.

Some of these delayed reactions can easily go unnoticed and not correlated to food because it seems to have nothing to do with the inside mechanisms of the body. For example, back to the chemistry analogy: Many people eat too many acidic foods. Eating too great a quantity of acidic foods can cause inflammatory illnesses like arthritis, eczema, aches in the joints, acne and other skin troubles. But because these seemingly have nothing directly related to the digestive system, the intake of food and how the body metabolizes it is often overlooked.

This is often overlooked, but is one of the most important factors of food. We are well aware that food is a physical substance, working to feed a physical body, but what is less discussed is that the body is also a body of energy, really, physically, and scientifically. As its cells spin, it creates a frequency. That frequency is energy. It would make sense then, to examine the energetic components of food as well. It would also make sense to understand that the more processed a food is the less natural energetic vibration a food possesses. This is often called a "dead food".

In contrast, one can eat fresh, real, whole, raw foods, or even juicing, and the effects are well noticed in a short amount of time, that the person feels alive and vibrant. These fresh whole unprocessed foods are called "live foods" and the energetic structure of the molecules themselves is entirely different than those that have been processed, stored in plastic, cans, and boxes, sat under fluorescent lights in a holding warehouse and then transported. It is not a stretch to imagine that the food would vibrate differently, with less matching frequencies of the body.

One has often heard that eating foods fresh from the garden, or within 15 minutes of juicing, or in sprouting are the healthiest options. This is because the food has fresh been plucked at the peak of its growth, where the food is most alive, containing the most nutrients, and having been recently in the energy of the earth itself. As a magnetic structure, the earth's energy itself is very powerful. Imagine the powerful energy that transfers from the earth to the food.

One can consume typical and conventionally processed foods, but by keeping it in balance with fresh natural earth grown and unprocessed foods, they still can maintain health in the physical body.

The more fresh foods containing high energy, the more optimally energized the body will be.

Kept this simple, understanding how to eat can be simple. However, because we have made our lives not simple, filled with expectation and time commitment, and the various other hosts of reasons that have separated us from our relationship with food, we have gotten off balance. This imbalance of course is going to demonstrate to us that the right fuel was not received and what we call "symptoms" will be evident. This is NOT the evidence of disease (yet), but the evidence that something necessary has not been received. And now in order to reduce or remove the unhappy result, instead of getting back into alignment with our relationship with food where we could identify the needs of the body, care for the provision of our food and how it's prepared, allowing that food to produce for our bodies, we hold tight to our schedules and fears and we search for anything and everything to remedy it, from drugs to specified fad diets.

Fad Diets

Fad diets are all part of the disconnected system that works like a machine to keep the vicious cycle working. They are a temporary fix, blaming the food itself as the reason for our trouble, avoiding all together the human alterations that changed the food, and most certainly avoiding true knowledge for a long maintaining balanced health with food.

Books have talked about individual foods or nutrients and they become a fad, or a particular diet plan , but rarely have I seen the basic simple functions of food. Instead, a new celebrity plan, a new food grown in the amazon is discovered, or new research is unveiled which explores "new knowledge" about a certain food. A fad diet does not work in the long term, is too radical and is not sustainable throughout life. Why they are successful in their following, however, is due to the fact that since its origination, people have used food for connection. Fads help a person to feel like they have a definition for themselves, that they fit somewhere. The current wellness trend is to "fit in" with the latest fad, even though this does not increase the relationship to, or give a real reason for adopting the new concepts.

It is less important in my mind, to have a LABEL, i.e. "I am vegan" than it is to answer the call of what the body needs in its service at the time. For example, I have been what others would term "vegetarian", "vegan", "grain free", "gluten free", but the most important thing to remember is that it is not about the label, which we use to simply identify ourselves, as it is to recognize what the body is telling us. Our body needs shift and so will our particular nutrient intake. In some people, the identification with a certain dietary lifestyle is freeing, but in others restriction of a certain diet only adds to the poor relationship with food that they already have. This phenomena is part of the reason why this book has a sister sequel, "Beyond the Plate", so that the deeper subconscious triggers can be worked with. What I propose in this book is not a new fad diet, but an explanation of function.

Special Diets for Healing

As a health practitioner, I can definitely agree that specified diets need to be used as a therapy for a period of time to help bring the body back into wellness. However, little effort is then paid to how to eat long term. Also, an understanding of how to eat in the first place needs to be taught so that we have the best chance of NOT experiencing dis-ease. In my experience with people, nutrition only becomes valuable once disease is present, missing the whole point of nourishment, which is as FUEL, not only as a REMEDY after the fact.

It is not acceptable to bounce back and forth from illness to specified diet, only to return to an illness-creating style of eating once again. True education of food and what it does for the body must be learned. The most important lesson to understand is that the function of the foods have not changed! It's like energy: it changes and transmutes, but it's basically the same as it ebbs and flows, depending on the nutrients available during its growth, but the function of the food still hasn't changed. It may have been produced poorly and/or altered in its processing, or grown in poor soil, but still the function of the food has not changed. What processing and conventional preparation DOES change is whether or not the food is living and actively available in service to us, or if it is a dead food, stripped of its value to us nutritionally and energetically.

It is important at this time that we go further into the difference between a living food and a dead food. A dead food is any food that has been cooked, preserved, or tampered with in any way that destroys some or all of the original vitamin, minerals, and enzymes contained in the food. This means any food not in its natural state. Anything cooked in a microwave is a dead food. After 10 seconds, all living enzymes in the food are gone. The enzymes are the part of the food that help our bodies to break the food down so that we can use it.

Living foods are foods that come to us as grown by nature. The foods that have the power to give us the most nourishment are those that are as close to nature as possible. If we CAN get natural foods, it is in the physical body's best interest to use them in preference to the unnatural dead foods.

Which brings us to our first of our four daily habits to dramatically empower your health outcome….the 5 Questions to Ask Before You Eat Anything!

Clean Your Plate

-7-

The 5 Questions To Ask
Before Eating ANYTHING

Here's what is true, no matter WHAT food belief set you follow. As we learned, foods have a FUNCTION, and PROPERTIES that are logical to learn if you want the right tools for the job. Understanding this puts you in the driver's seat no matter who or what is trying to feed you misinformation about your food and your options.

We discussed earlier what "food" is and and what is the right fuel for the job. If you look at the function chart, each function has food that are natural, real, and plant based. The section that the human body should be consuming the most of is the Eliminator category. Eating a good portion of your diet from the Eliminator category leads to a more alkaline, ph balanced, oxygen-rich (read: less cancer promoting), functional healthy body. Our 7D Nourishment principles will teach more about this balance in the next few chapters..

So in order, to see if a food product answers to the functions and principles we've discussed, the following questions can be asked to each and every thing you are preparing to consume:

1. Can I find it in nature?(or what is its natural state?)
2. Can I eat it immediately?
3. Does it need to be altered before I can eat it?
4. If I do alter it, does it change the health, value, and/or function of the food?
5. How does my body FEEL eating it?

If you cannot answer yes to the first two, chances are good that the nutritional value or function of the food changes. It does not mean that these foods can NEVER be eaten, but it does mean that there might be a warning to consume them consciously and within balance.

For example, an apple CAN be found in nature; it CAN be eaten immediately, it DOES NOT need to be altered before it is safe to eat. Foods of this variety can be eaten often, and easily.

An apple CAN be found in nature; it CAN be eaten immediately; it DOES NOT need to be altered, however it CAN BE. If I DO alter it, it DOES change the health and value of it as it reduces enzymes and possibly some of the nutritional content. So we would eat this less often as it's not in its natural state.

Rice CAN be found in nature; it CAN not be eaten immediately as it needs to be cooked first to reduce lectins, which means it needs to be altered. Altering it by cooking it makes it more digestible to the body, but as it cannot be eaten immediately in its natural state, you will want to eat in balance with those that can.

A cow CAN be found in nature, it CANNOT be eaten immediately, it DOES need to be altered before eating it. The fact that it CANNOT be eaten in its natural state is a warning sign for us to eat it in balance, if at all, with those that CAN be eaten in their natural state.

When you look at the variety of packaged conveniences on the shelf, it is very difficult to tell WHAT its natural state even was to begin with!

Question number five is commonly a very overlooked one. It seems we have created a disconnect with our bodies and our food. We discuss this more in the sister book, "Beyond the Plate". For now it is valuable for us to understand that food is not something that comes in and goes out without touching or making an impact on every part of the body. Food we bring in is fuel for our body's use. It is there to serve the body's needs. It it not meant to be the emotional support system we have created food to be, the feel good supplier, or the blame, curse or answer to all our problems. Plain and simple, food is to fuel the body so it can function. Our bodies will tell us a lot about how it perceives the food if we just listen to the signs it is giving us:

- Do you feel tired after eating it?
- Do you get itchy, antsy, or tense?
- Does your heart beat faster?
- Do you feel guilty?
- Do you hurt? Does it cause inflammation?
- Do you get congested? Stuffy nose? Runny nose?
- Does your skin itch or trigger eczema?
- Do you get a headache?
- If you picture yourself eating something, how can you imagine you will FEEL upon eating it?

The body talks through symptoms. It is important to listen.

Keep in mind, the questions are only a guidepost. In fact, they work the best for those that are following strictly a vegan, vegetarian or completely plant based diet, however as you can see, I find they still bring a lot of value to all options one is determining to ingest, to consider the proper amount and frequency.

Used at each meal, these questions will naturally bring you more awareness over how many enzyme rich foods you are consuming and how many cooked, altered, dead and possibly inappropriate foods you are consuming. This awareness will bring about more of a plant based focus, as sometimes we are simply unaware of how many dead or altered foods make up our diet.

Apply these rules to conventional packaged and processed "foods" and you will see, yet again, how they can hardly be called foods at all. You will certainly be able to see how they are not designed to be the right fuel for the body.

Eating fresh foods is essential to the functioning of the body. They are the original "fast food".

Clean Your Plate

-8-

THE 6 WORDS TO REMEMBER TO MAKE MEAL PLANNING FAST, HEALTHY, AND EASY:

FRESH FRIDGE FORMULAS FOR FAST FOOD

Welcome to The Garden of Eatin'

I fully believe we need to look to nature and copy it , because it has the answers. I highly recommend watching the series "Back to Eden Gardening" with Paul Gautschi. The concepts of living and working your own garden are inspiring through his work. If you don't yet garden your own fresh food, you can still use what is available to you through a community garden, a CSA(community supported agriculture), a local farmer or gardener, healthy markets, farmers markets, and more. This is my method of using what nature provides.

Fresh Fridge Formulas are not the ONLY way you can follow a healthy diet based in nourishment, it is merely a simple formula based option that can make getting started super easy. It is also a great way to encourage raw food eating, which is rich in natural living enzymes. This ensures you are getting a good portion of your food containing the natural food digesting compounds essential for proper digestion, and you don't even have to make the decision to become a "raw foodie"; it's already included in our Fresh Fridge plan.

Essentially, Fresh Fridge is a way of planning your week's meals with most of it prepared and ready for you to simply throw together. The fridge is stocked with fresh, cut, washed, and prepared fruit and vegetables, along with cooked and ready rice, beans, pastas, lentils, legumes, quinoa, and grains.

Formulas are prepared for you that are easy to follow to make a healthy plant based fast food breakfast smoothie, and lunch plate. This makes up your "70%" portion of 7D Nourishment. See how easy that is?

Then, your evening meal consists of anything you want, either:
* A vegetarian or vegan meal
* A meat based meal served with 2 sides of vegetables, prepared any way you like
*A meal containing grains and meat
* The food you love and don't want to give up
* This even allows for your party food, your weekend food, your guilty pleasures, at least as a baby step until you decide you don't desire them any longer.

I know, much is said about the evening meal being the larger meal. You can easily adjust your "30%" in various ways. I personally place it at the evening meal because that is when most families gather together, it is the most social time for eating unhealthier varieties of food; this way you can still participate. Since it often contains sluggish comfort foods, they leave a full and happy feeling before bed. The key is: don't starve and save up until your 30% meal and then binge on everything in sight. No matter when you eat your 30% meal, the day still is based on a 70/30 balance vegetation:convention. More will be explained in the next chapter.

Either way, if your total intake of food is 70% plant based and 30% meat, grain, or conventional the day is now much more proportionate and balanced for health.

Creating a fresh fridge is an excellent way to shake up your kitchen culture to encourage success in your health empowering diet. DrFoodie.live has resources and recipes to help you. Simply type in "7D"or "fresh fridge" in the website's search bar.

What is a Fresh Fridge?

A Fresh Fridge is a plant dedicated fridge. It contains fresh and healthy foods at the ready. Containers are filled with fresh foods, washed, cut and readied to make consumption and preparation easier. Staples like rice, beans, quinoa and pasta are pre-cooked and stored, ready to be used in the week, making lunch meals a snap, and making incorporating plant based foods a breeze. In the pantry, wraps or tortillas can be stored.

Having a fresh fridge is more appetizing and appealing to the eye if fresh foods are ready, it makes the brain more inclined to crave them. For those organized eaters, you will love how clean, vibrant and organized it looks, all of which makes one feel healthier just for having it available. Don't believe me? How do you feel in a cluttered room?

Creating a Fresh Fridge

Why? Why would you want to do this? Well, if you have chronic disease, symptoms, or extra weight, you want to take a look.

If you've wondered about being a vegan or a vegetarian but don't want to "give everything up", you want to take a look.

If you have dietary restrictions due to to nutritional illnesses, you want to take a look.

If you are unhappy with life, wish you had more self will, willpower, or self discipline, you want to take a look.

If you are tired of paying too much for groceries, you want to take a look.

If you just don't know how to navigate a healthy diet, you want to take a look.

If you are confused with fad diets and biases, you want to take a look.

Creating a Fresh fridge:

* It will encourage you to eat more vegetables and fruits

* It will encourage you to put your money where you want your body to be

* If it's there and ready, you're going to eat it, because we eat what's available

* It will teach your kids how to eat better

* It's cleaner

* Easier to prepare, easy and efficient through the week

* Less time consuming to prepare and clean up each meal

* Easier cleanup - no grease and messy pans

* Clean eating for your body

* Weight loss, as well as HEALTH GAIN, which is most important

* Reduce risk of chronic disease

* Feel better

* Better for the earth and the environment

* Cheaper - on the body, and on the pocketbook, ESPECIALLY if they come from a garden or farmers market, friend's garden, or CSA share!

How to Do It:

First: FILL YOUR FRIDGE - The FRESH FRIDGE Approach:

If you fill your fridge at the beginning of each week with fruits and veg, make it a challenge to eat them up before the week is through. Each week fill it with different varieties of produce. If they are prepared and cut the more likely you and your family will grab and eat them. The more likely you will add them to everything else.   If they are taking up your fridge space and you've spent money on them, the greater the chance that you will eat them.

For each person, plan enough fruit and veg for:

3 fruit servings a day

Lunch salads with 7 vegetables options in them daily

2 sides of vegetables at every supper

Frozen fruit for daily Breakfast Smoothies

Plus, you can create your weeks according to "theme", and choose produce accordingly. For example, have a mexican themed week and select veg that go better with tacos, burritos, taco salad, etc. Red, green, yellow, and orange peppers, jalapenos, rutabaga, lettuces, onions, tomatoes, cilantro, olives, avocado, hot sauce, etc. would be good staples for this theme.

Or Chinese theme and choose bamboo shoots, water chestnuts, celery, sprouts, shredded carrots, broccoli, snow pea pods, etc.

Follow the Fresh Fridge Formulas infographics at the end of the chapter for help with how to combine for a meal.

That's so much produce! Won't it all go to waste?

Not if you're eating healthy, it won't. If you're still trying to put into your belly all your other foods and you're eating them first, then probably. This is the point where you must ask yourself, "How badly do I want (fill in weight loss goal, health goal, body image goal, etc)"?

What if you didn't eat them all? What if the week ends, it's time to refresh your Fresh Fridge and you still have some left over. Don't throw them out!

* Greens can be frozen to add to smoothies, soups, casseroles, juices

* Fruits can be frozen to add to smoothies

* Fruits can also be dehydrated and make dried fruit. Fruit can be pureed and poured onto a dehydrating liner to make fruit leather.

* Bananas can be frozen to make banana ice cream

* Herbs can be dried to be used as spice or frozen and used in casseroles and soups

* Many can be used to grow the next...for example, celery can grow a new celery shoot, garlic can grow more garlic, potato eyes can grow more potatoes, etc!

* When in doubt, COMPOST! At least it will CREATE dirt to grow the next batch in!

Second, Prepare the Plant Based Proteins and Grains:

Prepare the bases to go along with your fresh produce. For example, boil beans, noodles, quinoa, and rice. Keep in containers in your fridge so that it's easy to pull meals together.

Third, Plan the Evening Meals

While your Fresh Fridge accommodates Breakfast, Lunch, and Snacking and will add to your evening meal, this is where you will need to plan your evening meal and add the necessary items to your grocery list.

Ideas for Creating Meals With Your Veg:

Recipes are available on Drfoodie.live for more suggestions.

*Make a lentil and vegetable soup to eat throughout the week so it's easy to have a well balanced, nutritious meal available in minutes, when you can't prep a Fresh Fridge Lunch.

* Every week, I make 1 soup that can be eaten throughout the week, or frozen in single servings and kept for much later on, or a quick meal when needed.

* Black Bean and Veg Soup, chock full of beans and Fresh Fridge leftover veg!

* Vegan burritos with rice, beans, all kinds of veg(and a side of burger for the carnivores)

* Taco night with all the vegetable fixings and herbs and a variety of beans and meats for meat eaters

* Stir fry and rice

* Spring rolls, with thai peanut sauce my favorite!

* Vegetable spiralized noodles with sauces, try this one with mushroom alfredo sauce!

* How about Asian flare with cabbage slaw, brown rice, edamame and peanut sauce!

* Add some Mexican flavor with romaine and peppers, brown rice, black beans, salsa and guacamole!

* How about spinach, quinoa, white beans, and marinara!

* Make it mediterranean with cucumbers and tomatoes, quinoa, garbanzos, and hummus!

Here's What's So Cool About It:
* It follows Food Fx(functional eating) and 7D Nourishment (70%plant based, 30%animal/grain/conventional product as desired) and the Law of Nourishment for balanced eating.

* Even if you don't like this all the time, but a week here and there, will benefit.

* You can easily follow the Fresh Fridge Formulas for easy fast food healthy eating to get a good breakfast and lunch, then healthy snacks through the day with the fresh produce in your Fresh Fridge and then eat what you want for

supper

* Statistics show the majority of the problem is through the day when we're out and about, and late night eating, or the type of eating we do when we're being social, so this is acknowledged through this lifestyle of eating. The times you are generally social and doing the worst eating is already accounted for, and plans for it so there's ZERO GUILT.

* For weekends, we eat "weekend food", which means we generally do what the crowd we are with does. If we are at home, we eat leftovers and get the fridge read for the next week. We choose the new produce and get it prepped. We cook new batches of rice, noodles, dried beans and lentils and put them in the fridge ready to go. We bake and eat whatever appeals to us on the weekends, especially if we have swapped some of our 30% suppers into Fresh Fridge 70% meals.

A Word on Snacking

The "reason" for snacking would be for someone who needs additional nutrient intake, is in a progressive and active healing plan, or who has specific blood sugar needs that requires snacking frequently (however, these people should be balancing their body systems at the same time for whole health improvement, which is sadly, often lacking). Snacking gets us into trouble when we use it for comfort, boredom, or any other misplaced emotion.

What is commonly overlooked is that sometimes the feeling of hunger is actually dehydration. The simple fix is to drink an 8 oz glass of water and wait 20 minutes,then see if you are still hungry.

One of the other culprits is that the body could be lacking in nutrients that it desperately needs and is trying to get your attention. Awareness must be present so as to determine if there is a valid reason the body wants the food it is wanting. In working with clients over the years, I have learned that sometimes the body may be dehydrated, but specifically it may be "electrolyte" dehydrated, meaning it doesn't have the proper electrical balance of sodium and potassium necessary in the cells to create the electrical energy the mitochondria rely on. Making sure to have proper electrolyte balance through foods like celery(with the leaves), leafy greens and juicing, or consuming coconut water can have a drastic effect on the body, causing it to use more of it's nutrients and feel more energy and less cravings.

Another useful and intentional purpose for snacking may be so that a person is holding sugar longer, in order to provide energy to systems, or so that proteins ride on sugars in order to decrease up and down swings for mood or hormones.

Snacking provides the fuel for your body to keep going. However, the science behind it is that if you are on weight rebalancing plan, you generally do not want to snack, forcing your body to get its energy by burning fat.

Snacking is generally out of habit, rather than hunger, and often the perceived hunger is actually due to hydration. It might be worth the trial to drink a glass of water and get yourself occupied in a task that is fun and useful to your transformation to redirect your habit.

One problem we see with snacking is not only that it is generally a habit rather than a bodily need, but that the snacks are "treats": processed, garbage junk food that the body does NOT need to refuel with, but that you are using out of habit, comfort, or any other false reason that doesn't bring you to health. An ACTUAL snack's purpose to refuel the body would be something that brings the body value, like fruits, vegetables, nuts, or seeds. Even in a person that has been medically determined to need frequent meals throughout the day, the key word still is "meal". It is not an opportunity to load up on junk. It is still intended to be a well balanced actual meal of nourishment.

Basically, whatever the train of thought, "snacking" is largely misunderstood, ill-applied, and inappropriate to the body's needs.

Take some time to observe your snacking: why you are conceptually choosing to snack, what you are feeling, and what you are choosing as your "snack". Understanding these concepts and learning the habits of your mind will go a long way towards understanding your choices. Our relationship to food is one of the biggest factors to consider when we're having misalignment and imbalance.

Breakfast: Starting Your Day Without Caffeine

Think coffee is the only way to get you jump started in the morning? Here's why this goes against the Nourishment Principles for your body.

Why did we EVER get in this habit? And if you pay attention, it's not just one coffee in the morning to get things going....it's multiple....darker....and throughout the day. Sure it gets you going, but at what cost?

First of all, I have an issue with what we're all avoiding. The fact that we need this jumpstart says quite a bit about the life we are living. Why are we living in such a way that life is a drudgery we have to jumpstart to make it through? That's the first problem, and the first resolution, by the way.

As far as what happens when you drink that coffee, It's all about brain chemistry, but instead of working with and nourishing the brain, you are manipulating and fooling the nerves...bad idea in my book, folks. Pure and simple, here's what's up in summary. A substance called Adenosine is created in the brain, naturally. It again, naturally and innately intelligently, binds to receptors made just for it....Adenosine Receptors. This binding slows down nerve cells and causes drowsiness. This activity also causes blood vessels to dilate, in order to get more oxygen to the brain during sleeping. It's how sleep works.

However, when you ingest coffee, the CAFFEINE LOOKS like Adenosine to a nerve cell, and so now the caffeine binds to the Adenosine Receptors. Except, it DOES NOT slow down the nerve cell. It constricts the blood vessels, providing LESS oxygen, and speeds UP the nerve cells because this is now a threat to the adrenal glands, our "fight or flight" glands. Thinking we are in danger, the adrenal glands push out chemical messengers that speed everything up...in order to get us out of danger. This is why you are instantly awake, because the body has told you to be ready for action. Does that sound healthy to you? By the way, adenosine also has a major effect on Dopamine, sound familiar? It's HUGELY related to feelings of wellness...or DEPRESSION, a commonly diagnosed condition in today's age.

When you ingest caffeine, your heart speeds up, your blood pressure rises, your airway opens up to start inhaling more oxygen (for survival), your muscles tense up ready for action that your body didn't naturally prepare itself for and is the reason you can suddenly feel like running a mile, your liver purges sugar into the bloodstream for extra energy (you know, because you just downed coffee, and didn't fuel your body with any breakfast, sound familiar?)This has a huge thwarting effect on your metabolism by the way. Weight gain, anyone?

Plus, once that coffee wears off, you hit that proverbial low....and you reach for the pot again.

In a SUPPORTIVE way to work with the body:

1. To get it moving is first and foremost...create a life you LOVE that you can't wait to wake up to!

2. Waking up and BREATHING MORE through awareness like meditation or yoga, and also breathing more simply because you are awake and moving more, particularly if you do say ten minutes of exercise.

3. Just like breathing more, there are herbs that are food, fuel, and fortifiers to the body as NOURISHMENT, (not like caffeine which acts more like a drug...forceful and abrupt, without the body's say). Herbs were MADE to assist bodily function. Where caffeine constricts the blood vessels, providing less oxygen to the brain resulting in chemical warriors to come in and fight for you, an herb like Ginkgo Biloba, for example, dilates the blood vessels, allowing the brain to receive more oxygen, not out of panic I might remind you. This natural increase of blood flow to the brain creates mental alertness and focus.

4. Let lemon water be the first thing you put into your body. Lemon boosts energy levels without the caffeine crash. When the negative ions in the lemon hits your digestive system it increases energy levels. If drunk first thing, it helps purge the liver, and a sluggish liver leads to a sluggish body so it only makes sense to stimulate the liver, correct? Plus, lemon is in juice form and is more readily bioavailable to the body so it can start nourishing and energizing the body immediately on contact. Basically, lemon does what caffeine does, but not induced by a hormonal state of forceful panic and fight, but because it

is assisting natural functioning.

5. B Vitamins - They help take the food you put into the body and reap the energy out of it. So hello, eating breakfast(which most coffee drinkers skip in favor of their cup of jo) in general would be a start, but drinking a greens rich smoothie, or green juice would be even better.

6. Breakfast - the nourishing kind, which provides fuel for your body to operate off of. And no swinging through the drive through either. At least grab a protein smoothie alongside your green juice. If you set your kitchen up right to accommodate this, it can be just as fast. Prepare for your success by having the right tools and making it easy!

7. Lastly, and most importantly, if you need something to keep you going throughout the day, you might not be doing things right for yourself. It's no different than needing a drug or alcohol to "get you over the hump". Relying on ANYTHING as a NEED is harmful to your mental, emotional and physical state. Be responsible to examine what your life's cues are telling you and create the life you love.

I believe coffee is an herbal plant medicine….but that it was not intended to be ingested, only used effectively in other methods like coffee enema therapies.

A breakfast plan following formulas for health, like the Fresh Fridge Formulas are a healthier, balanced wy to start the day. As stated before, Fresh Fridge Formulas for Fast Food are not the only way to follow 7D Nourishment, but it is an easy way to start. As long as you understand the Food Fx, the functions of food, you will be well on your way to a more balanced diet.

Look to the following pages for infographics for the Breakfast and Lunch Fast Fridge formulas.

Amanda E. Soulvay Plevell, PhD

7D NOURISHMENT

FRESH FRIDGE FORMULA
BREAKFAST SMOOTHIE

Consuming quality nourishment from plant based sources for 70% of your daily intake can be key in reducing inflammation and your risk of chronic disease.

1 CHOOSE ELIMINATORS -
51 cup, fresh or frozen -

trawberries Mango
Blueberries Pineapple
Raspberries Cherries
Blackberries Orange Melon

Eliminator

2 CHOOSE YOUR LIQUID
1-2 cups (depending on desired thickness)

Almond milk
Hemp milk
Cashew milk
Macadamia milk
Soy milk
Coconut Milk
Orange juice
Cranberry juice
Green juice
Water

Builder
and/or
Eliminators

3 Add Builders

2 scoops protein powder
½ cup yogurt
2 Tbsp Chia seeds(also lubricator and fiber)
2 Tbsp Flax meal(also lubricator and fiber)

Builders
Add 1/2 frozen banana for thickness

Sources:
Not a medical doctor. For educational purposes only.
www.drlandielive.com

7D NOURISHMENT

FRESH FRIDGE FORMULA LUNCH

Consuming quality nourishment from plant based sources for 70% of your daily intake can be key in reducing inflammation and your risk of chronic disease.

1

Eliminator and/or Congestor

CHOOSE YOUR BASE

Rice, Vegetable noodles made with your spiralizer (zucchini, sweet potato, etc), Mixed Greens, Sprouts, Spinach, Vegetables (raw, steamed, boiled, baked) Baked potato, Salad, Vegetable mix (cucumber, carrots, radish, daikon, green onion) Pasta, Lettuce leaf, Tortillas Spring roll wrap, Nori wrap, Quinoa, Lentils Brown, Rice

2

Builder and/or Eliminators

FILL IT UP!

Greens - sprouts, herbs, cabbage, romaine, spinach, mustard greens, turnip greens, collard greens

Veggies - Peppers, Cucumbers, Celery, Daikon, Onions, Carrots

Grains - Quinoa, millet, amaranth, brown rice

Beans and legumes - Black beans, kidney beans, pinto beans, lentils, chick peas, hummus

3

Lubricator

Top With Flavor

Sauces: hummus, guacamole, salsa, pesto, marinara, hot sauce, olives, olive tapenade, Avocado
Dressings: Lemon squeeze, Lime squeeze, Apple cider vinegar, Tahini, Miso dressing, cashew dressing
Oils: Olive oil, avocado, sunflower, grapeseed
Nuts or seeds: Pumpkin seeds, Sunflower seeds, Chia, Flax, Hemp Seeds

Making Adjustments

Baby steps are OKAY! Following the Fresh Fridge Suggestions and formulas are a great place to start and can also be used as a foundation if you need to start a little slower. Either way, it's going to make vegetation more of a central part of your diet, where it needs to be.

As your body adjusts, you will eventually feel cleaner, healthier, and lighter. This feeling makes it much easier as you won't tend to crave the same meat proteins and grain products that you usually do. As you go along, you also won't feel so hungry. The balanced fresh foods will start to feel filling and satisfying, so I definitely encourage keeping on following the Fresh Fridge Formulas while your body makes the transition.

In the meantime, perhaps you want to follow the formulas, but ALSO add a small portion of meat or grain alongside. Either way, it will keep these portion sizes down, while increasing your plant based intake. The trick is, to think about the fruits and vegetables FIRST, adding the grain and meat secondary, as needed.

As another option, if you continue to eat grain and meat products at all meals, you might consider at least beginning to create balance with a functional ORDER to your diet:

Step 1. ELIMINATOR – If you eat raw eliminators first, you prepare the body and its digestive juices and digestive process to accept the more difficult to digest foods that are coming.

Step 2. BUILDER – Eat your builder portion second, now that the body is prepared to digest it.

Step 3. ELIMINATOR – You can eat as many eliminators as you want. You can have them cooked, steamed, or raw, or a combination of all three.

Step 4. CONGESTOR – If you are STILL hungry, then allow yourself a congestor whether it's bread or dessert, just keep in mind how big the serving size should be.

(YOU WOULD EAT LUBRICATORS AS NEEDED WITHIN THE STEPS)

What is most important is that you keep the Food Functions in mind and plan accordingly. Fresh Fridge Formulas simply make it easy by taking away the planning, speeding up prep and clean up times, include essential enzymes through raw fruits and vegetables and ensures balanced structure during your day. If you are doing Fresh Fridge Formulas, you are ALREADY following 7D Nourishment and Food Functional balance.

Drfoodie.live has a RESET 30 day program in which Fresh Fridge Formulas are planned out for you daily, as well as evening meals, and coincides with conceptual growth and personal transformation activities as well. We'll discuss more on this in the chapters to come, but you can also check it out at www.drfoodie.live. and find RESET 30 Day in the main menu.

-9-

7D NOURISHMENT

Fresh Fridge Formulas are simply one way to easily implement the practice of 7D Nourishment. This means that 70% of your intake comes from plant sources and 30% from meats, grains, or conventional foods, (all being inflammatory foods)if at all. This is more in alignment with how the body is designed to nourish itself, thus preventing disease, inflammation, and symptoms.

Much of society's ills can be attributed to overdone and imbalanced eating, particularly of improper foods. The number of diseases that are nutritionally related and the number of people suffering from them is staggering!

---

*It is estimated that 678,000 deaths each year
are nutrition and obesity related.*

That does not even account for the number of diseases that are caused in part or in whole by improper diet.

It would make sense that since our food is what becomes our body that we would both prevent disease process and assist it's healing with food.

The belief is held strongly that many of these diseases can be completely prevented, or at least moderated with diet, so it would make sense to understand the properties of food that keep our systems functioning well.

When we study the functions of the body, eat foods that function those functions, and do that in balance, the body is more inclined towards healthy manifestations.

Much of the current American diet consists of far greater protein and bread carbs than are required or are even healthy for a human body.

Ed Cederquist, of the popular monaker, Bistro MD mentions one particular risk with our confusion over and addictive love for grain carbs stating that, "Higher intakes of carbohydrates, such as a diet that provides greater than 65% of energy in the form of calories from solely carbohydrates are associated with increased triglyceride levels in the bloodstream, as well as reduced HDL cholesterol, which is 'good' cholesterol in the body. This puts individuals consuming too many carbohydrates at a greater risk for the development of atherosclerosis and heart disease."

7D is a balanced style of nourishment in which the intention is in accordance with innate needs and original functional purpose of a body. Basically, feeding the body with the particular functions and properties that go to serve the individual functioning parts and systems of the body.

7D Nourishment is DrFoodie's planned program for a healthy dietary lifestyle. It was developed after studying multiple beliefs and methodologies of nutrition ultimately reaching the conclusion that not only does the nutrition that is on your plate matter, but that maximizing the body's NOURISHMENT once it is inside your body is even greater.

The 7D Nourishment method allows for the greatest bioavailability from the food's you eat, promotes the best digestion possible, focuses on balance with an understanding to the Functions of Food, encourages support of the body's overall functioning with the least amount of inflammation possible, all because the body's originative functions are taken into account, as well as an understanding of the functions of food and why we were designed to eat them.

Whether a person identifies as meat eater, a vegan or vegetarian, the diet is easy to adapt, and does not focus on restriction or complete removal or avoidance of any one particular food, but is designed to have the majority of the diet be made up of the foods that are necessary to the body's natural mechanical systems and their ability to function properly.

7D stands for "70", as in 70%. 70% of the diet comes from at least 70% plant based sources, and 30% in which grain, animal proteins, and or conventional foods are allowed, if at all. Those that identify as vegan or vegetarian simply would not add the animal proteins or products derived from other beings. For those that have not chosen that particular lifestyle, 70% plant based nourishment brings the amount of animal protein and bread carbs down to a more balanced level, still allowing the foods that contain the important eliminative functions and anti-inflammatory properties to lead the way.

The goal of this particular discussion is not to determine whether or not one should be vegan or a meat eater, or to judge any particular belief set, but to help all bodies be able to nourish themselves in balance according to functions of food, and in accordance with the functions of the body. Please understand this is not a judgement or an instruction on what "should" be, merely a well strategized plan for those wishing to incorporate a more health promoting diet. Either choice still includes more vegetation, which ultimately restores balance to the diet.

This nourishment plan is also easy to make gluten free, and grain free as desired for certain diet related healing protocols, as it is meant to be a low inflammatory diet. I personally choose, and coach my clients, to take into consideration health as a whole and do not choose to use my 30% times for unhealthy fats, processed foods, and refined sugars, but to supply my body with the healthiest level and quality of real food I can.

What Does This Look Like In Real Life?

This could look like across the 7 day week, up to 3 days are allowed to have animal product meals. Some would translate this at 21 meals a week = 7 meals that can be meat and bread carbs, or 1 meal a day, which works particularly well for those just beginning this style of nourishment.

However, it is this author's opinion that eating meat daily does not allow the body ample time to recover from the inflammation and acidity that comes along with consuming animal products. It is my particular preference in coaching meat eating individuals to choose 3 days a week in which you will allow animal products if desired. This way, there is time in between the 30%

meals for restoration. It is up to each individual how many meals on those days will contain animal products, according to personal preference and belief. Those that choose no animal products can simply keep all of their meals plant based, but would still be observant keeping other other conventional and grain foods to 30%.

Through my online toolkit, DrFoodie.live, I work to make following 7D Nourishment easy. A 30 day RESET Lifestyle diet can be found there, as well as charts, articles, and exercises to help you be successful.

-10-

IT'S TIME FOR A RESET

Here's How the RESET Works....

If you're feeling like it's time for a reset, this is a great place to begin! Learning something new takes time and dedication....and a plan doesn't hurt either!

Many come because they just feel like they're getting nowhere with their health. Some come because they don't know where to START with their health.

I'll tell you where...it ALWAYS comes down to food and what you feed your physical body with. That's what DrFoodie is all about: the FOOD (or poison) you nourish your body with and the mental food or poison you nourish your mind and soul with!

It takes a reset to get back on track and the fastest way to improve BOTH your body and your mind/spirit/soul is to feel better with food! Then you have the energy to do the other important work to attract your best self yet.

With ANY healing in any dimension of your life, feeling better is going to increase the wealthy health in ALL areas of life.

So Let's Begin with FOOD! It's a great way to practice and develop self will, self control, and self discipline, which is super important for every other goal orientation you may create with yourself.

With me so far?

Here we go....

How this works so that you can make this the most successful reset. This reset posts lifestyle plans every day for your use for 30 days. Each post is chock full of links to recipes, articles, and exercises all over DrFoodie.live's online toolkit, giving you maximum education right at your fingertips. These get "added to your cart" and then downloaded to your email inbox. Most of them are free, some are of varying amounts, and NONE of them are an obligation to you to purchase, whatsoever! They are there to help YOU! Even if everything in your cart is free, you still "check out". Following this you will receive the downloads. We do this so that the best information is going to people that have real intention on healing and improving their lives. It helps us keep track of who has had access to what, so that we don't repeat ourselves or so that if we do work with you in the future we don't waste your time with what you've already had.

This way, you can get the basics for a doable reset, yet not be overwhelmed by too much information unless you request it. Keep it simple. Don't get overwhelmed. Just follow the reset and ignore the links if you need to. If you find you have an interest in more information through a link, follow it and check it out. If it's for you, add it. If it's not, simply come back to it later. This is meant to help YOU! The great thing is that you can store all of your email downloads in an email folder on your computer and come back to them again and again!

Let's begin...

Time to reset! This dietary plan is designed to reset your taste buds so not only are the more healthy foods less offensive to you, but you'll actually start to develop a taste for them. This includes the absence of ALL processed foods, junk food, refined sugar and sugar substitutes, dairy, gluten, and alcohol. Why were some of these even classified to be called something that should go into our bodies in the first place?

The RESET 30 Day follows a clean eating diet with the 7D Nourishment as a guide. This means RESET is going to teach you to practice eating 70% of your diet from plants and vegetation, and 30% from grains,meat and animal products if you choose it. The RESET is made so that people in all areas of readiness can benefit. All meals you will find to be vegan or vegetarian. The idea is that all day will be plant and vegetable based. The 30% percent portion comes in at the end of the day meal, where you are allowed a meat option. DrFoodie writes vegan or vegetarian meal plans because I believe it's harder to come up with plant based meals and I'm sure you already have meat and conventional meals you already love you can add in on your own. If you choose to eat meat, then 1 meal containing meat per day, along with a balance to servings of vegetables, is planned per day. This also works for those trying to conform to a grain restricted diet. In this case your 30% meal (1 meal a day) could be the meal in which you add a grain side.

The RESET follows the Fresh Fridge Formulas, wherein, the breakfast uses a smoothie formula, and the lunch uses a vegetation formula. Then, the evening meal you can choose to follow the vegan/veg meal suggestion DrFoodie lists, or you can choose one of your conventional meals to enjoy. Over time, what most people have discovered is that they crave the meat and grains less and less, and move to "30%" being only 3 times a week do they indulge in conventional meals. Soon, many find that they make the switch to a complete plant based diet. The point is that ANY of these steps is an improvement over the current diet, so allow yourself to grow and take its baby steps.

The closer you stay to whole foods in the RESET, the faster your body will respond to good nutrition.

-11-

8 DIMENSIONS OF WELLNESS

I believe that people do often times feel imprisoned by their health or lack of it. It's a fact that food has to have an impact on your health, AND on your illness. We also believe people want to get out of the feeling of imprisonment. True health cannot happen without a strategy for the mind. If there isn't balance in all Dimensions of Wellness, the physical balance proper eating creates will only be short lived.

This author personally believes that the health of the body, mind, and soul is what creates the manifestation of wellness in all areas of the body, what we call the "8 Dimensions of Wellness", that EACH of those dimensions has to be balanced and healthy if we want to feel a free life, one that we enjoy.

We believe that in a holistic mindset, that ALL of these dimensions need to be examined and fulfilled. These dimensions are:

1. Spiritual
2. Physical
3. Financial
4. Relational
5. Occupational
6. Intellectual
7. Environmental
8. Emotional

I fully believe that it starts in how you feel IN THE BODY, because if you feel sick and unwell, chances are good you are not going to want to work on any of the other dimensions. Your food intake is something you CAN take charge of and start anew EVERY DAY. If you've ever been focused on healing or learning ANYTHING new, you know how important it is to find teachers you trust, with experience, and educational materials that really make a difference. You also know you have to want it. You have to be committed to yourself, your education and your future. We know this to be true as for over 12 years, DrFoodie has mentored health seekers searching for a happy healthy life, whether for their own personal health and happiness, or to be trained to teach it to others.

We've learned during this time that the student has to be ready. And learning has to be habitual, daily, and routine in order to be successful. They say it takes nearly 30 days of doing something EVERY DAY for a habit to change.

Think back to grade school when you were learning to read. EVERY DAY you would be learning skills, exercises, and pieces of the puzzle until you had the whole thing down. And you DIDN'T even realize you were learning! Because it was fun and small parts of the whole were broken down DAILY until reading just became a successful part of your everyday life.

Changing your health through diet has to be a decision EVERY DAY, EVERY MEAL in order for that habit, and your health, to change.

But in doing so, we fervently and strongly believe that YOU CAN have freedom - whether that freedom is in health, finances, work, or all of the above. But it takes DAILY steps, and the purposeful intention of daily commitment to new actions and thought processes. That's why we have created an online toolkit, where you can access purposeful and intentive lessons articles and exercises so you can keep growing and share it with others!

We want to help those committed to growth, life, and health so that we can:

* get exclusive information to you DAILY

* to make sure you have enough information for all dimensions to learn new habits of living, so that you are DAILY living differently

* Get enough information to you so that you can see noticeable change in your life.

Conventional understandings, thought processes, commonly held beliefs of our world and society's way of living are NOT going to get you there!

The RESET 30 Day Lifestyle Challenge

In the last couple of chapters, you learned the trueest daily plan for getting started on a new eating lifestyle, during which you will change your daily habits, learn WHY you're doing it, sample new recipes, and identify the Core Concepts that could be keeping you stuck in a state of stagnation.

You'll be able to use these 30 days to completely transform the direction of your life and who you want to be by daily taking steps towards it. You'll be able to get in the habit of health, with a plan laid out for you while you learn what works for you. Not only does this transform the direction of your eating habits, but the manifestation of your health, which ultimately impacts the other dimensions of the 8 Dimensions of Wellness - your wealth, your relationships, your work, your finances, and every other area that you choose.

Consider the Rewards

Just think where you could be 30 days from now, what you could look like, feel like, and think like. When you commit to the RESET 30 Day, you are committing to better yourself, take your power back, cast your vote, and be better for yourself and the people you love. By waking up each morning and daily living the habit it takes to make change, you will develop discipline, self will, and determination - character traits of which who knows where else they may take you?

Combined with our concepting work that goes along with each day, you'll be developing success habits and the mindset needed to improve your life.

By asking yourself the 5 questions before you eat anything, committing to your meals using the 6 Words to make fresh easy (Fresh Fridge Formulas for Fast Food), and by following the 7D Nourishment principles, you will daily be enhancing the wellness of all 8 Dimensions. You'll be generating more energy, creating more control over your health, and empowering yourself to take bold movements for change. Who knows what will happen when you access the power of YOU?

People have done this month over and over until it sticks, and you are welcome to do it as often as you need. You also have all of the information in the DrFoodie.live online toolkit, as well as the community on our Facebook page: cleanyourplate5678.

Steps to Begin the RESET 30 Day Challenge

1. Go to www.cleanyourplatebook.com and and get started on "Day 1: Beginning Your Reset", which links to the following days. You will also see links to helpful tools and downloads to track your progress and grow as you go.

2. Get an accountability partner. Send someone a message to join you in empowering the decisions over their health. In fact, send them the link listed in #1. It will cost them nothing and you will be teaming up with someone who has the same commitment as you to improve their life. Don't WAIT until you have a partner, start NOW and make them want what you have! Don't delay in improving your life.

3. Set a date that you will begin your 30 day Challenge and mark it in your calendar.

4. Join the facebook community at facebook.com/cleanyourplate5678

Conclusion

It's never too late to determine
to be who you want to become.

No matter what's happened to you in the past, where you have been, what you look like, what you USED to look like, what you USED to be able to do, it is never too late to improve your life. It is what we are here to do! To be happy, to live our personal Greatness in such a way that it can't help but to spill over and help someone else too! Today, and every day after, determine to live your best self and take the steps that are bound to improve every area of your life.

Get your RESET kit today at www.cleanyourplatebook.com, join the Facebook community, and share what you are learning with others. Have fun having kitchen parties! Get creative with your fresh foods and share them with others so they can experience a clean plate too! Who knows whose life you will help change.

If there's anything I can do to help you and your group to be successful, don't hesitate to email me at info@cleanyourplatebook.com. You can book me to speak and educate others on what you are doing to dramatically and boldly put the power of your health back into your hands. To do this or order group bulk discounts, send an email to sales@cleanyourplatebook.com.

One final thing...Let's Spill This Out and Impact Others

Can I be so bold as to ask you to help me change the world, one plate at a time? If this book and information on our website have helped you, would you please share it with others? Let them borrow your copy or give it as a gift. Especially to those you know are suffering, the gift of true health can make a big difference in someone's life. If you believe as I do that it's time to stop being imprisoned in our bodies and minds, please share this book, spread the word, and share the love. Thank you!

Clean Your Plate

Breakfast Smoothie Sample Recipes

MVP Daily Smoothie

Combine and blend until smooth:

1/2 cup frozen strawberries

1/2 cup frozen mango

1/2 frozen banana

1 tbsp frozen OJ concentrate

1-2 cups almond, coconut or hemp milk (depending on how thick you like it)

1 tbsp chia seed

1 tbsp flax seed, ground

1 scoop vanilla or berry flavor pea protein powder

Great "Beet"-ing Heart Breakfast Smoothie

Combine and blend until smooth:

1 small red beet (if using a vitamix or very good blender, use a raw beet. If using a poor quality blender, slightly steam the beet first)

1 half of a lemon, squeezed

1 tsp grated fresh ginger

1/2 c frozen raspberries

1/2 c frozen strawberries

1/2 cup cold water

1 scoop plain, berry, or vanilla flavored protein powder

(Try also adding a handful of goji berries)

Chocolate Hazelnut Smoothie

Combine and blend until smooth:

1 frozen banana

1 scoop chocolate flavored protein powder

dash of vanilla extract

1 cup of almond milk

1/4 c raw hazelnuts(or try cashews or macadamia nuts to shake it up)

Mint "Ice Cream" Chocolate Smoothie

1/2 c coconut yogurt or coconut cream from can

1 frozen banana

1 scoop of a Greens powder (I use Nutrition Dynamics Dynamic Greens Mint for the mint flavor, but you can add a 5 drops of peppermint essential oil along with 1 scoop of plain greens powder as well.)

3 pieces of cooked broccoli (your kids will never know the difference)

1 scoop chocolate protein powder (I use Ultra Meal by Nutrition Dynamics)

Blend well and drink.

Berry Fine Smoothie

1 cup frozen strawberries

1 cup almond milk

1 cup frozen spinach

1 scoop berry flavored protein powder

More breakfast smoothie and vegan/vegetarian recipes available at DrFoodie.live.

Clean Your Plate

References

Food Babe. "Is Coconut Oil Healthy? The Controversy Explained." Food Babe, 7 Feb. 2018, foodbabe.com/coconut-oil-healthy-controversy-explained/.

"Our Food Story | Fresh and Delicious Weight Loss Meals." *BistroMD*, www.bistromd.com/our-food-story.

"Annual American Fitness Index Expands to Rank 100 Cities Arlington, Va. Is New #1 'Fit City'." William Lyon Homes Announces Agreement to Acquire RSI Communities, a Southern California and Texas Based Homebuilder | Business Wire, 15 May 2018, www.businesswire.com/news/home/20180515005131/en/Annual-American-Fitness-Index-Expands-Rank-100.

"CONCEPT-THERAPY." CONCEPT-THERAPY, concept-therapy.org/.

"Intro." Dr. Thurman Fleet, www.drthurmanfleet.com/.

"Home." Dr. Jason Lupkes, DC, www.zonehealer.com/.

"Vegan Protein." Vinchay Fit cards, www.pinterest.com.

Zieve, D (2009, May 2). In Protein in Diet: MedlinePlus Medical Encyclopedia. http://www.nlm.nih.gov/medlineplus/ency/article/002467.htm

"Building Complete Proteins from Nuts, Grains and Legumes /
Nutrition / Proteins." / Nutrition,
www.fitday.com/fitness-articles/nutrition/proteins/building-complete
-proteins-from-nuts-grains-and-legumes.html.

Brain, Marshall, et al. "How Caffeine Works." HowStuffWorks
Science, HowStuffWorks, 1 Apr. 2000,
science.howstuffworks.com/caffeine4.htm.

I highly recommend studying the principles discovered in "Back To
Eden Gardening" with Paul Gautschi and play your part in
cooperating with nature.

Resources and recipes are available on drfoodie.live
Also will you find there information on the "Clean Your Plate"
Experience, where you can attend intensive workshops and
experience a diet following Clean Your Plate Principles.

ABOUT THE AUTHOR

Amanda Plevell is living proof that every single one of us lives inside a miraculous body. That no matter the adversity that we face, we can still create the most extraordinary life we can dream up!

Amanda faced a multiple disease - snowball effect in her health over a 7 year time span. After facing Arterial Hemorrhage, Ulcerative Colitis, Crohn's disease, thyroid disorder, 5 miscarriages, 1 stillborn birth, and 1 D&C, the health dilemmas only continued. Steroid Induced Myopathy lead to experiencing life in a wheelchair and a year of recovery including relearning to walk and rebuild a body. The situation was grave and serious, yet Amanda defied the "impossible" and using God, truth in food, a tribe of healers, mentors, and friends, has gone on to heal entirely without medications. She allowed the self to go back to nature's perfect function through the use of food and finding herself, which became the tagline for her online wellness company: DrFoodie.live.

During this time, she also completed her Doctorate in Clinical Natural Medicine/Naturopathy and her PhD in Natural Medicine from the New Eden School of Clinical Natural Health in Indiana, following her Bachelor's training in Education, Counseling, and Certification as Natural Health Professional. She earned a Diploma in Biochemical Nutrition from the College of Natural Medicine and went on to begin the WellClinic Community Wellness Centers, The Natural Source Companies for Wellness, has written over 30 self help books and now works with people all around the world to improve their whole being.

She is intent on teaching and living a Consciousness Lifestyle with intent on expanding global good through natural functional wellness, lifestyle by intentional design, and Concept Pathology.

She is a dedicated trainer, speaker, community wellness and teen advocate, developing programs to support growth and to encourage each individual she encounters to Be The Change.

Clean Your Plate

Amanda E. Soulvay Plevell, PhD

**Other Books by
Amanda E. Soulvay Plevell
Available on Amazon**

The Answer

The Real Heal: Genesis Vs. Genetics: Why Science Can Never Divorce
Energy From Healing

Your Final Forty

Be The Change

The Genesis Code

Successfully Conditioned Teen

The Healed, the Healer, and the Healing: CPT

5+1=0

The Love Letters

Successfully Conditioned Kids

Tribe

Intuitive Unschooling

Your Great Big Beautiful Life

Your Great Big Beautiful Life Companion Book

Soul Colored Love

Anxiety Turnaround

Clean Your Plate

Dragonfly Journal

Gifts of a Dragonfly

I am Success

Mandala Coloring Book

My Book of Firsts

No Grain No Pain

Questions for Answers

Success Conditioning Work It Out Book

Success Conditioning Journal

Successful Relationships

The Energy of Divorce

Instructional Book Club Kits and discounted bulk quantities available by contacting sales@cleanyourplatebook.com

Amanda E. Soulvay Plevell, PhD

The Clean Your Plate Experience

The Clean Your Plate Experience is an intensive week long and weekend retreats to take a step out of your normal life and really apply yourself to principles of higher learning and evolution. All meals are provided and follow the principles presented in "Clean Your Plate".

It's an opportunity to meet yourself, and other like minded individuals, apply a lifestyle of healthy eating, learn principles of evolution and discover the Greatness Within each of us.

Be sure to like our Facebook page www.facebook.com/cleanyourplate5678 to join the community all over the world for your daily Clean Your Plate Experience.

Clean Your Plate

Amanda E. Soulvay Plevell, PhD

Pre-Order Now!

"Cleaning" Your Plate is just the beginning! A healthy relationship with food, dealing with emotional blocks, limiting concepts and beliefs, and learning to love yourself as nature in perfection is extremely important.

Don't stop with the end of this book!

Having a healthy relationship with food, your concepts about it and yourself are the second huge portion of a healthy lifestyle with food. Identify what concepts may be holding you back in the sequel to "Clean Your Plate"

Flight Plan Publishing is currently accepting pre-orders
for the sequel: "Beyond the plate"

Get your copy now at DrFoodie.live!

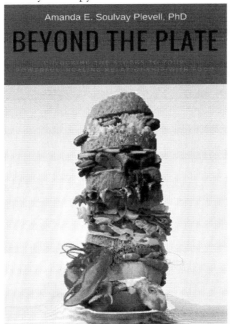

Clean Your Plate

Notes

Amanda E. Soulvay Plevell, PhD

Notes

Made in the USA
Columbia, SC
27 June 2018